THE FRAGRANT ART OF
AROMATHERAPY

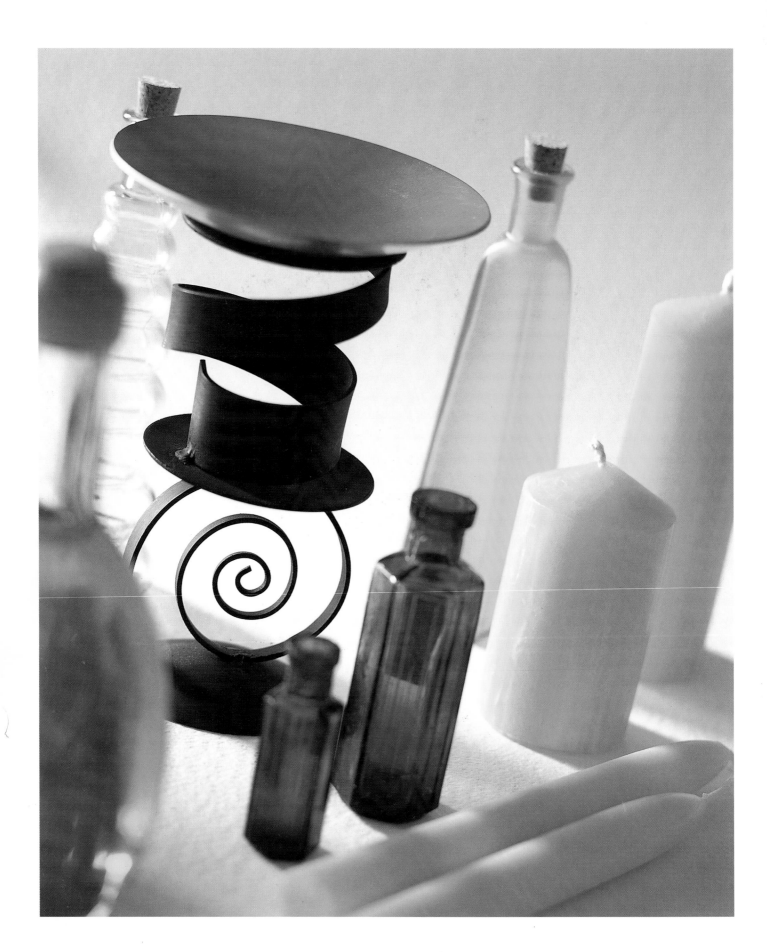

THE FRAGRANT ART OF
AROMATHERAPY

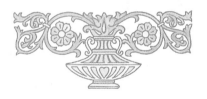

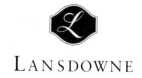

Lansdowne

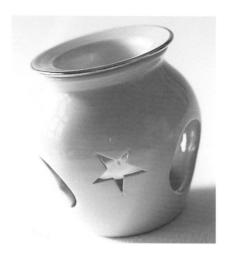

Contents

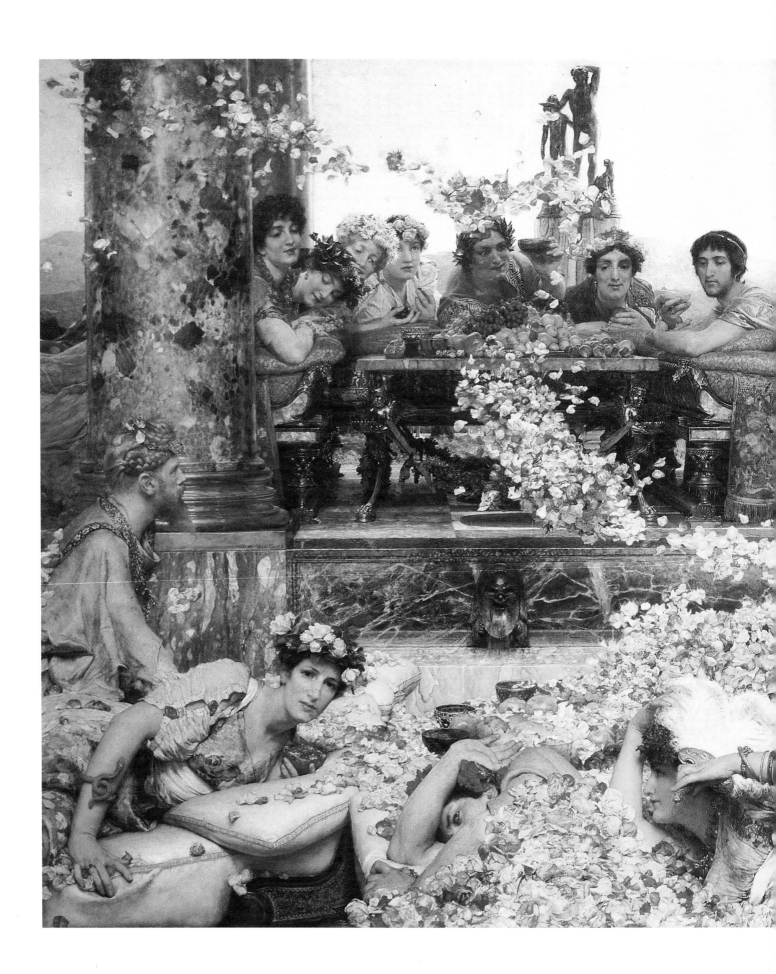

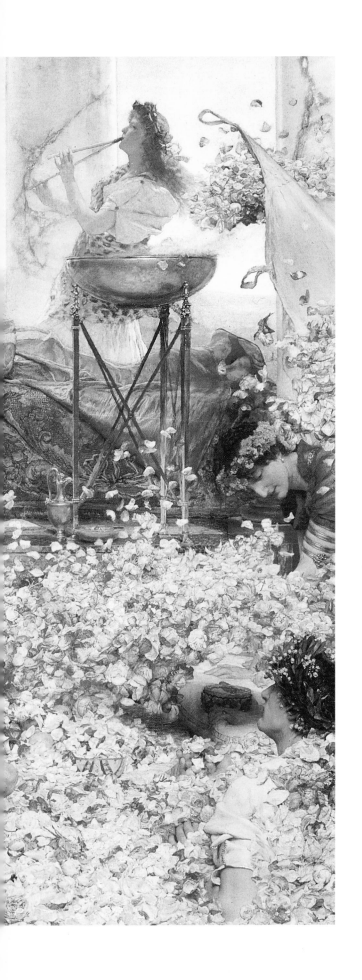

Introduction to an Ancient Art

*Essential oils
are pure concentrated
extracts from selected plants.
They are revered
both for their fragrance and
their therapeutic value.
It is the use of these essential oils —
in vaporizers, atomizers,
baths and light bulb rings,
as compresses or inhalations,
in massage oils or cosmetics —
that is known as the practice
of aromatherapy.*

Records of oils essential to the body, mind, and emotions may date back to the time of legend, but their beneficial effects are certainly not a myth.

The Ancient Egyptians were thought to have known about the benefits of essential oils, and it is said that Cleopatra had her clothes, her rooms, and the sails of her ships permeated with the oils of jasmine and rose.

Hippocrates, the Greek physician known as the father of modern medicine, apparently accepted the connection between essential oils and their therapeutic use. He prescribed aromatic baths and scented massages and recommended certain oils because they offered protection against contagious diseases.

In the Middle Ages, in particular, monks cultivated herbs and discovered many of their restorative properties. They were among the first to distill precious plant essences, carefully blending them into liqueurs to be administered to patients.

The modern-day interest in oils began in the 1920s when a French chemist, René-Maurice Gattefosse, was making fragrances. While working in his laboratory he burnt his arm, and immediately plunged it into a jug of lavender oil for relief. To his amazement the pain was less than he expected, the blistering was greatly reduced, and the healing process sped up. Gattefosse was so impressed he spent the rest of his life researching the healing properties of essential oils and he coined the term "aromatherapy". Scientists have confirmed that many oils have important chemical properties that are aids to healing.

Essential oils should never be confused with fragrant oils, perfume oils, or aromatic oils, which are not pure extracts and do not have the same therapeutic value. And, despite the name, essential oils should not be thought of as "oily".

Aromatherapy is not limited only to the sense of smell, although this does play a part. The sense of smell is a powerful vehicle that can affect the inner balance of the body, and your subconscious. Think of how the smell of baking can lift your spirits and bring back childhood memories. Or how unpleasant smells can make you retch. The fragrance of essential oils works on this level, but it also has a deeper dimension.

The essential properties of the oil can also be absorbed via the hair follicles on the skin. These properties are then transported around the body and affect various organs and body systems. Aromatherapists use the oils singly or in combination. They talk about "synergy", when the combination of the oils creates a chemical compound which is more powerful than the individual oils.

Aromatherapists can choose from about 300 essential oils that are now traded around the world. The oils are produced from all types, and parts, of plants — flowers, leaves, stalks, gums, seeds, and roots. To ensure the best quality, the plant must be picked at the optimum time; in the case of sandalwood, that means waiting 30 years until the tree has matured. This is the reason for the variation in price between different oils. Some oils are relatively easy to extract while others involve a very complex process or a relatively scarce supply of the plant itself.

Lavender oil is relatively simple and inexpensive to make.
Rose, however, is the queen of the oils and very expensive. It takes tens of
thousands of rose petals to produce just one small bottle of oil.

Professional aromatherapists can choose from about 300 essential oils that are now traded around the world. For home use, you would normally need no more than 30 of the most common and readily available oils and 10 or 12 oils should be sufficient for all the requirements of the average household (see the chapter The Essential Oils, pages 10–19, for suggestions). The oils are produced from all types, and parts, of plants — flowers, leaves, stalks, gums, seeds, and roots. To ensure the best quality, the plant must be picked at the optimum time; in the case of sandalwood, that means waiting 30 years until the tree has matured. This is one reason for the variation in price between different oils. Some oils are relatively easy to extract while others involve a very complex process, there may be a relatively scarce supply of the plant itself, or it is a low-yield plant and a large quantity of the plant is required in order to extract the oil. Petals from more than 30 roses are required to make just one drop of essential oil of rose, for example. Price is often comparable with quality and may be a good indicator of the purity of the essential oil. For the purpose of aromatherapy only the purest extracts can ensure the desired effect. Be sure to always buy authentic essential oils in air-tight, dark glass bottles from well-known and reliable distributors.

Particular essential oils are believed to have special properties, ranging from antiseptic to aphrodisiac effects. Some promote relaxation and a general feeling of balance and harmony, others stimulate and rejuvenate. All can encourage a feeling of well-being and can be used to treat or prevent health problems, or simply to create a mood and pamper your senses. For stress and stress-related health problems, aromatherapy is an ideal treatment; the beneficial aromas can sooth frazzled nerves, quiet an over-stimulated mind, release tensions in the muscles, and relax the body.

Different essential oils may be prescribed by a professional aromatherapist for varying conditions. For example, chamomile is useful for tension and irritability, rosemary is good for poor circulation and fatigue, and lavender is an all-purpose oil for many ailments from burns to headaches to insomnia.

Generally, it is safe to use essential oils at home, although there are some oils you should use with caution and some oils you should not use if pregnant (see contra-indications given in the chapter The Essential Oils, pages 10–19), and you should consult your medical practitioner and a qualified aromatherapist if you have any serious health problems.

The Essential Oils

There are about 300 essential oils used by professional aromatherapists. This chapter contains 29 of the most popular oils and details some of their extraordinary properties so that you can make the best use of them at home.

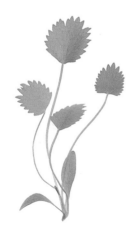

Basil

Botanical name
Ocimum basilicum

Extraction
The oil is obtained from the flowering tops and leaves.

Description and history
Cultivated for at least 4000 years, basil has had a somewhat contradictory reputation. It was native to India — where it was a sacred herb, believed to protect against evil — and spread from there to Ancient Greece, where it became a symbol of hostility and insanity. Basil appears to have reached Europe by the mid-16th century. It was used both as a strewing herb and as a medicine (primarily for settling an upset stomach), and the oil was used to scent snuff.

Properties
Digestive • respiratory • soothing • calming • relaxing to muscles • head-clearing • uplifting • clarifying • aphrodisiac • mentally stimulating • aid to concentration • refreshing • useful for soothing skin abrasions

Caution
Avoid use during pregnancy.

Bergamot

Botanical name
Citrus bergamia

Extraction
The oil is derived from the fresh ripe peel of the bergamot orange after the juice has been extracted.

Description and history
Bergamot essential oil blends well with other oils to enhance their aroma and is most commonly used in commercial perfume manufacturing, being a key ingredient of eau de Cologne. It is a powerful antiseptic and may be diluted for treating skin or scalp conditions and for dressing wounds. It has a natural deodorizing effect, both as a breath freshener and as a personal deodorant.
Depression and anxiety are effectively treated with this refreshing oil.

Properties
Respiratory • uplifting • clarifying • antiseptic • digestive • treatment for skin and hair • refreshing

Caution
This oil is phototoxic; do not use on the skin in sunlight.

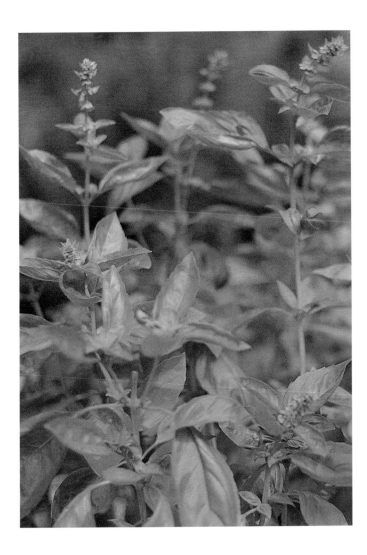

Bay

Botanical name
Laurus nobilis

Extraction
The oil is distilled from the leaves and berries of bay.

Description and history
According to classical legend, the bay tree was sacred to Apollo, the god of medicine. The aromatic oil has long been used as a soothing rub for arthritis and rheumatism, and an aromatherapist may prescribe it to relieve earache or to lower blood pressure.

Properties
Soothing • antibacterial • circulatory • anti-inflammatory • relaxing

Caution
Avoid external use of bay if you have extremely sensitive skin, as it may provoke a rash.

Chamomile

Botanical name
Matricaria chamomilla (German), Anthemis nobilis (Roman)

Extraction
The oil is distilled from the plant's flowering tops.

Description and history
There are many different types of chamomile, which has long been cultivated as a medicinal herb. The oils of German and Roman chamomile share similar soothing properties. Chamomile oil became so popular in Germany as a medicine that it was known as "alles zutraut", meaning "capable of anything". It has been variously prescribed to speed healing, calm inflammation and allergies, and treat burns, bruises, earache, neuralgia, abscesses, and toothache. The fragrance has a definite calming effect — a steam inhalation can assuage insomnia and hysteria. It is also a useful oil for natural beauty care, especially as a hair conditioner, and is a very effective treatment for skin disorders.

Properties
Soothing • mildly antiseptic • analgesic • calming • relaxing to muscles • digestive • refreshing • balancing for the female system

Caution
Should not be used in the early months of pregnancy.

Cedarwood

Botanical name
Juniper virginiana

Extraction
The oil is distilled from the wood of the tree.

Description and history
One of the oldest known essential oils, cedarwood was an important ingredient in the medicine, cosmetics, and perfumery of the ancient Egyptians. The strong balsam-like fragrance of cedarwood essential oil makes it useful as an all-round tonic and stimulant. It can hence be used to treat problems concerned with a sluggish system, particularly respiratory and skin complaints. Cedarwood is thought to possess aphrodisiac properties, presumably because of its exhilarating scent.

Properties
Antiseptic • digestive • astringent • skin-toning • calming • aphrodisiac • harmonizing • strengthening • sedative • soothing

Caution
Avoid use during pregnancy.

Clary sage

Botanical name
Salvia sclarea

Extraction
The oil is obtained from the flowering tops of the plant via steam distillation.

Description and history
Although related, this is a completely different oil from common sage (*Salvia officinalis*). Along with bergamot oil, clary sage oil is a key ingredient of eau de Cologne and lavender toilet water. Clary sage has an astringent and tonic action, helping to stimulate the digestion, and calm fevers, and produces a wonderfully cooling effect on the skin. For this reason, it may be included in cosmetic preparations to cleanse the skin, particularly dry or sensitive skin. The oil has a marked relaxing effect and may be used to treat stress, high blood pressure, depression, and anxiety. It is also excellent for the female system.

Properties
Soothing • anti-inflammatory • calming • relaxing • skin-toning • astringent • warming • uplifting • euphoria-producing

Caution
Avoid use during pregnancy.

Clove

Botanical name
Carophyllus aromaticus

Extraction
Cloves are actually the unexpanded flower buds of the clove tree.

Description and history
Centuries before Christ, envoys to the Han court of China held clove oil in their mouths to freshen their breath during audiences with the emperor. Later, the oil was to serve as a protective agent against the bubonic plague. Clove oil is one of the most effective antiseptics known, good for treating infections, especially colds and flu. It is often an ingredient in commercially available mouthwashes and digestive tonics and will bring a welcome numbness if applied topically for toothache or sore gums.

Properties
Antiseptic • antispasmodic • slightly aphrodisiac • analgesic • carminative • digestive • nervine • respiratory • warming

Caution
Avoid use during pregnancy.

Cypress

Botanical name
Cupressus sempervirens

Extraction
The oil is distilled from the tree's leaves, cones, and flowers.

Description and history
The resinous, woody oil contains several strongly aromatic principles which work together as an effective tonic for nervous disorders, by acting as a sedative on the nervous and respiratory systems. The oil is a common ingredient in many commercial preparations used for the treatment of colds, bronchitis, or flu (try a few drops on a pillow or handkerchief to relieve nasal congestion). Cypress oil is also a powerful astringent useful for healing wounds and balancing problem skin, or for circulatory problems. The oil is also a good natural deodorant.

Properties
Balancing to the female system • stimulating • circulatory • respiratory • decongestive • head-clearing • antispasmodic • gently diuretic • refreshing • relaxing • astringent

Caution
Avoid the use of cypress oil if you suffer from high blood pressure.

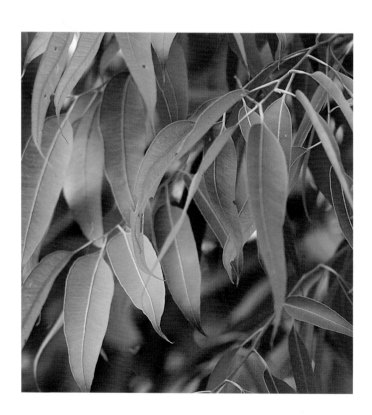

Eucalytpus

Botanical name

Eucalyptus globulus

Extraction

The oil is distilled from the leaves of the tree.

Description and history

Eucalypts are among the most aromatic plants in the world, and the sharply scented oil has powerful healing, disinfectant, and antiseptic uses. Well known for its use in inhalants for treating respiratory conditions, the oil is also useful for wounds and insect bites. Cooling to the body, a compress made from a cool dilution of eucalyptus oil can relieve fever and skin irritations. Used in vaporizers or room sprays, the oil helps cleanse and disinfect the air.

Properties

Anti-inflammatory • antispasmodic • analgesic • refreshing • stimulating • uplifting • invigorating • respiratory • head-clearing • decongestive • antiseptic • cooling • cleansing

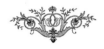

Frankincense

Botanical name

Buswellia thurifera

Extraction

The oil is distilled from the resin in the bark.

Description and history

Frankincense was one of the most highly prized substances of the ancient world. In Ancient Egypt, frankincense was much prized as a skin tonic. Today, this beautifully scented essential oil is recognized for its decidedly restorative action, making it ideal for more mature skin. It is used to treat respiratory complaints, for it has the effect of slowing and regulating breathing. This calming property makes it a good nerve tonic and also a useful aid for meditation.

Properties

Nervine • respiratory • restorative • beneficial to the female system • rejuvenating • comforting • relaxing • soothing • fear-dispelling

Geranium

Botanical name

Pelargonium graveolens

Extraction

The essential oil of geranium is mostly obtained from the leaves, via steam distillation.

Description and history

One of the most widely used essential oils in perfumery and cosmetic production, geranium is acclaimed by aromatherapists as a good "all-rounder". It may be prescribed for emotional disorders, to treat skin conditions, and as an insect repellent. Geranium oil is astringent and refreshing, and its rich sweet aroma makes it a popular choice for massage treatments and footbaths. Its principal effect is on the blood, making it a wonderful relief to tired and aching limbs. Use it in a vaporizer to treat respiratory complaints, or as a gargle to treat a sore throat. A balancing oil, it is invaluable for skin care, for the female system (especially for new mothers), and for harmonizing the emotions.

Properties

Antiseptic • antidepressant • anti-inflammatory • diuretic • balancing • skin toning • warming • refreshing • relaxing • harmonizing

Jasmine

Botanical name

Jasminum grandiflorum

Extraction

The essential oil is extracted from the petals through the time-consuming process of enfleurage, which makes it one of the most costly oils.

Description and history

Cleopatra used oil of jasmine to woo Mark Antony, and today it is an ingredient of many fine perfumes. The oil is highly esteemed for treating problems of the nervous system, dispersing depression, tension, listlessness, and fear. It is often included in natural skin care products for its smoothing and softening effect on skin, and is useful for preventing scarring by increasing the skin's elasticity.

Properties

Relaxing • uplifting • beneficial to the female system • strong sensual stimulant • soothing • confidence-building • aphrodisiac

Juniper

Botanical name

Juniperus communis

Extraction

The essential oil of juniper is made from the berries of the juniper plant.

Description and history

Known since ancient times for its antiseptic and diuretic qualities, juniper has a marked effect on the digestive system, the female system, and the circulatory system — whether used in a massage blend or prescribed orally. By association, problem skin can benefit from the oil. It serves as a useful general tonic — a few drops in a warm bathtub or in a massage oil is helpful in treating sleeplessness and stress.

Properties

Nervine • diuretic • analgesic • toning • cleansing • relaxing • balancing • refreshing • digestive • circulatory • appetite-stimulating • carminative • invigorating • relaxing to muscles

Essential oil of juniper shouldn't be confused with juniper oil which may be cheaper, but is less effective, and usually made from the leaves and twigs.

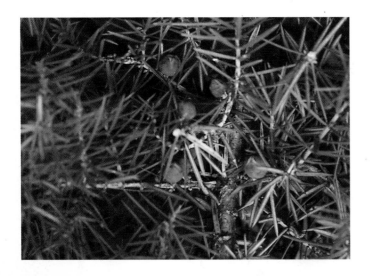

If you were to choose only one oil, it would have to be lavender. Safe to use even directly on the skin, its antiseptic and healing properties make it a must for the first-aid kit, and its soothing qualities help ease everything from headaches to emotional upheavals.

Lavender

Botanical name

Lavandula officinalis

Extraction

The oil is distilled from the flowers, leaves, and stems.

Description and history

Commercial perfume houses use essential oil of lavender as the basic ingredient of many fragrances. It is also the most widely used and versatile healing oil. Not only is it extremely effective, but it is also very easy to use and one of only two oils that can be safely applied undiluted to the skin (the other is tea tree). Lavender oil may be used with great success to treat skin disorders, preventing scarring and promoting rapid healing. It is also one of the stronger antiseptic oils and is included in a variety of cosmetic aids such as mouthwash, skin tonic, and eye-lotion, in addition to making a natural insect repellent. The oil provides a soothing rub for arthritis and rheumatism, a good inhalant for respiratory problems and fainting, and a relieving compress for headaches. The balancing properties of lavender can correct emotional problems and feelings of instability. Its calming effect will induce a restful sleep.

Properties

Head-clearing • respiratory • skin-healing • nervine • digestive • sedative • calming • balancing • analgesic • antiseptic • antibacterial • decongestant • antidepressant • refreshing • relaxing • soothing • relaxing to muscles

Lemon

Botanical name

Citrus limomum

Extraction

The oil is obtained from the rind of the fruit.

Description and history

This fresh, sharply aromatic oil is used to treat nausea and to stimulate the appetite. Use it also as a massage to aid circulation. The lemon's antiseptic properties are well respected, and make it effective in treating colds and sore throats and in controlling skin blemishes. The mild sedative action will reduce fever and ease indigestion. Most particularly, lemon oil helps to stimulate the body's own natural defences against infection. This oil may also be used as a natural cosmetic. It has a wonderful toning effect, and mild deodorizing properties, and will provide a gentle exfoliating action. Use it as a rinse or in a bathtub to lighten hair or skin, as a tooth cleanser, or in a cooling lotion to soothe sunburn.

Properties

Antiseptic • physically stimulating • skin tonic • astringent • antibacterial • diuretic • circulatory • refreshing • cooling • uplifting • stimulating • motivating

Caution

This oil can be phototoxic; avoid use on the skin in sunlight.

Marjoram

Botanical name

Origanum majorana

Extraction

The essential oil is extracted from the leaves and flowering tops of the plant by means of steam distillation.

Description and history

This strongly aromatic oil may be added to a base carrier oil and used as a gentle rub for muscular aches, bruises, sprains, and arthritic pain. It also has a very strong effect on the female system. It is the most strongly sedative of all essential oils and can quieten excessively heightened emotions and offer sleep to the insomniac, especially if enjoyed in a warming bath.

Properties

Antispasmodic • carminative • sedative • nervine • calming • relaxing to muscles • digestive • warming • fortifying • respiratory

Caution

Avoid use during pregnancy.

Myrrh

Botanical name

Commiphora myrrha

Extraction

The essential oil is distilled from the gum resin produced by the bark of a small Middle Eastern tree.

Description and history

The essential oil of myrrh is a highly aromatic oil with a deep golden appearance and a sweet, camphor-like scent. It has been used to treat and disinfect wounds and skin problems, and for digestive upsets. Myrrh oil may be used as an antiseptic gargle and is very useful for dental problems, hence its use in many toothpastes.

Properties

Healing • digestive • anti-inflammatory • respiratory • tonic • stimulating • antifungal • astringent • antiseptic • toning • strengthening • rejuvenating • expectorant

Caution

Avoid use during pregnancy.

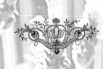

Neroli

Botanical name

Citrus aurantium

Extraction

Neroli essential oil is extracted from the orange blossom.

Description and history

It is popularly thought that this oil was named after the 16th century Italian Princess of Nerola, who used it extravagantly to scent her clothes and rooms. Neroli oil is extremely expensive, but the perfume is absolutely exquisite. It is much used in perfumery, notably in the production of eau de Cologne. Neroli makes a wonderful facial oil and massage blend, helping to regenerate skin cells and improve skin elasticity. It is one of the most suitable essential oils to use for nervous tension, insomnia, and stress-related illnesses, as it has a very positive calming influence on both mind and body. It is rumoured to have aphrodisiac properties, no doubt owing to its deeply relaxing effect and its enticing scent.

Properties

Antibacterial • calming • healing to the skin • circulatory • nervine • digestive • sedative • antidepressant • aphrodisiac • relaxing • fear-dispelling

Orange

Botanical name

Citrus aurantium (bitter orange)

Citrus sinensis (sweet orange)

Extraction

In contrast to neroli, both the sweet and bitter essential oils of orange are extracted from the peel of the fruit.

Description and history

The aroma of orange essential oil is deliciously fresh, which promotes a bright and sociable mood. Its light, tangy crispness makes it a delightful room freshener. Add it to your bathtub for instant refreshment. Being both refreshing and sedating, it is a wonderful remedy for depression, tension and stress. Like neroli, it also benefits the skin — particularly if dull and congested or troubled with cellulite. The oil is rich in Vitamin C, making it a good treatment for colds and flu.

Properties

Astringent • relaxing • refreshing • uplifting • antidepressant • digestive • antiseptic

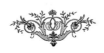

Patchouli

Botanical name

Pogostemon patchouli

Extraction

The oil is distilled from the dried branches of the bushy patchouli, a member of the lavender family, originating in Bengal, India.

Description and history

The oil has a strong and persistent smell and is often used as a fixative in commercial perfume production or to mask over-strong aromas in cosmetics. It is also an effective moth repellent. Patchouli oil is useful as an antiseptic, particularly as a first-aid treatment for minor burns, as it has an anti-inflammatory effect. The oil also works on irritated nerves, calming anxiety with its strongly earthy scent. Aphrodisiac powers are attributed to the sensual, musky aroma.

Properties

Anti-inflammatory • aphrodisiac • nervine • sedative • relaxing

Peppermint

Botanical name

Mentha piperita

Extraction

The oil is distilled from the leaves and flowering tips of the plants.

Description and history

Peppermint oil, particularly as an inhalation, relieves nausea and respiratory problems, and aids digestion. A gargle made with the oil will both assist these conditions, and freshen the breath. A mild washing water made by adding a few drops of peppermint oil to distilled water is a cooling lotion for those with sensitive skin. The cooling effect extends to the emotions, clearing the mind. Rats and mice detest the invigorating aroma, so rags soaked in peppermint oil are a very effective deterrent to vermin.

Properties

Digestive • carminative • respiratory • anti-inflammatory • balancing to the female system • cooling (and warming) • clearing • relaxing to muscles • refreshing

Pine

Botanical name

Pinus sylvestris

Extraction

Essential oil of pine is distilled from the resins and needles of pine trees, of which there are over 100 varieties.

Description and history

The clean, fresh smell of pine oil is a familiar, everyday aroma — it is used extensively in soaps and bath preparations, as well as household cleaning products, for both its scent and its antiseptic properties. Pine oil is a powerful antiseptic, probably best known for its effectiveness in treating infections of the respiratory system. The oil has a stimulating effect on the circulation, making it a warming rub for painful muscles. With this invigorating quality, pine oil will help to treat lethargy and listlessness.

Properties

Respiratory • antiseptic • nervine • stimulating • refreshing • invigorating • deodorizing

Caution

Pine oil should not be used by people with sensitive skin, as it may cause skin irritation.

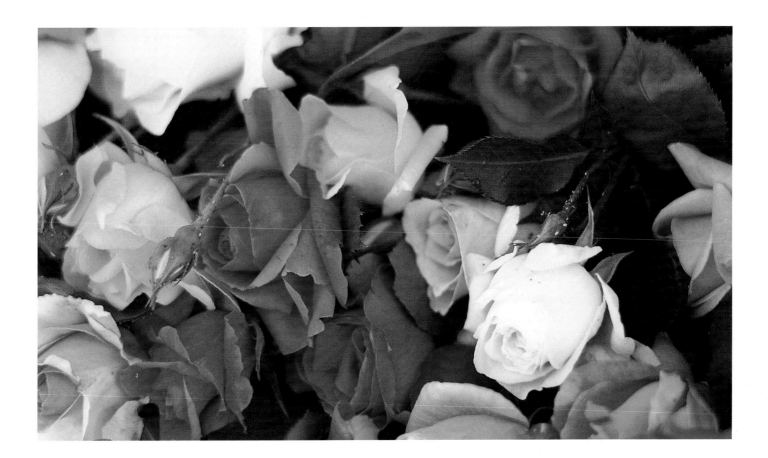

Rose

Botanical name

Rosa damascena (rose otto), Rosa centifolia (rose absolute)

Extraction

The "queen of essential oils" is one of the most prized and most valuable oils — it takes the petals of 30 damask roses to make one drop of rose otto essential oil.

Description and history

Rose oil is probably best loved for its marvellously feminine and sensual fragrance. Therapeutically, this scent has a potent antidepressant effect and may be used, via face and body massage, skin preparations, baths, or vaporizers, to treat nervousness, sadness, or long-term stress. Rose oil is often included in cosmetic creams for its refreshing, mildly tonic effect on sensitive skin. Diluted in distilled water, rose oil may be used in compresses for tired or inflamed eyes. The oil is also an excellent remedy for disorders of the female system.

Properties

Antibacterial • antiseptic • astringent • anti-inflammatory • antidepressant • digestive • confidence-building • sensual • aphrodisiac • balancing • relaxing • soothing

Rosemary

Botanical name

Rosemarinus officinalis

Extraction

Essential oil of rosemary is distilled from the flowering tops and leaves of the plant.

Description and history

Rosemary oil has been used in many preparations to ease the processes of ageing. It is recommended for hair care and as a scalp massage to prevent premature baldness. With its powerful aroma, rosemary oil is an effective inhalant and decongestant, and a strengthening massage rub for muscles. This is the most stimulating of oils, enhancing memory, concentration, and clear thinking.

Properties

Invigorating • digestive • nervine • respiratory • circulatory • muscular • uplifting • stimulating • refreshing • clarifying

Sage

Botanical name

Salvia officinalis

Extraction

Sage oil is still extracted from the plant's leaves using traditional methods that have changed little over the centuries. The leaves are spread out to dry naturally in the sun on racks before they are distilled. Accordingly, sage oil is often slightly more expensive than most other essential oils.

Description and history

Essential oil of sage has an astringent and cooling effect. It may be used as a blood cleanser, and to promote the appetite, cool fevers, ease headaches, and heal skin conditions or wounds. It may be used diluted in distilled water as a gargle and mouthwash. Sage oil is an extremely effective natural deodorant and antiperspirant, and can be burnt in a sick-room to help cleanse and purify the air. It was once widely used as a remedy for "the ague" or rheumatism, and massaging with it helps ease nervous and muscular tension or pain.

Properties

Diuretic • analgesic • antiseptic • decongestant • astringent • nervine • relaxing • refreshing • stimulating

Caution

Avoid use during pregnancy.

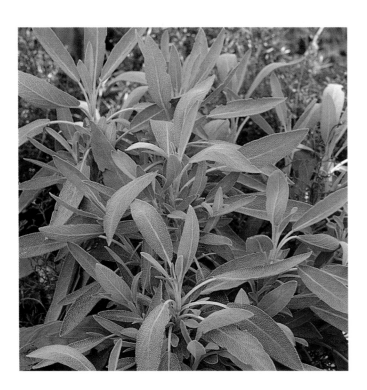

Worshippers in Indian temples covered their bodies in essential oil of sandalwood, rose, jasmine and narcissus. Sandalwood also blends well with neroli, basil and frankincense.

Sandalwood

Botanical name

Santalum album

Extraction

Essential oil of sandalwood is derived from the wood of the sandalwood tree, via steam distillation.

Description and history

This exotic essential oil captures the mystique of Asia, where it forms part of Ayurveda, the Indian system of healing. It is probably best known as an ingredient of perfumes and scented cosmetics, as an essence in its own right, as a complementary fragrance to most rose scents, or as a fixative. It also has preservative qualities, and helps to give creams and lotions a longer life. Sandalwood oil is an excellent facial oil, being particularly soothing and emollient for dry, or irritated and sensitive skin, as it helps cleanse, heal, and soften. This oil also has a potent calming effect on the nerves and digestive system, making it very helpful for an upset stomach. The rich, woody aroma provides a relaxing and supportive environment for meditation, and promotes confidence and well-being. If you are feeling cold, a few drops of sandalwood oil in a hot bath will leave you wonderfully warm.

Properties

Digestive • softening and healing to skin • antispasmodic • antidepressant • calming • relaxing • soothing • sedative • warming • confidence-building • grounding

Tea tree

Botanical name
Melaleuca alternifolia

Extraction
The oil is obtained from the leaves via steam distillation.

Description and history
The fresh, lemony scent of tea tree oil is very pleasant, having a marvellous cleansing and head-clearing effect. Tea tree oil is renowned as an antifungal and antiseptic treatment, and may be used directly to treat skin conditions and wounds, or as an inhalant to treat respiratory infections. Diluted and applied topically, it is very effective in correcting bacterial imbalances in the female system. Tea tree oil also serves as an efficient natural insect repellent, and is often included in cleansing preparations and insect collars for cats and dogs; the oil may be used in a vapourizer to repel mosquitoes.

Properties
Antiseptic • antifungal • digestive • healing to skin • antibacterial • respiratory • decongestive • strengthening to the immune system

Thyme

Botanical name
Thymus vulgaris

Extraction
Essential oil of thyme is obtained from the flowering tops of the plant via steam distillation.

Description and history
Thyme has long been used as an antiseptic, a decongestant, and a digestive aid, and for respiratory treatment. It is also said to retard hair loss. Diluted in distilled water, thyme oil is a good general tonic and assists the circulatory and immune systems. In vaporized form it fights infection. The oil is strengthening mentally and emotionally as well as physically. It is recommended for hangovers.

Properties
Antiseptic • disinfectant • circulatory • respiratory • nervine • stimulating • refreshing • cleansing and toning to skin • relaxing to muscles • strengthening to the immune system • fortifying

Caution
Avoid use during pregnancy.

Ylang ylang

Botanical name
Cananga odorata

Extraction
Essential oil of ylang ylang is extracted by steam distillation from the flowers of the tropical ylang ylang tree of Java, Indonesia, the Philippines, and Madagascar.

Description and history
The sweet, heady scent of ylang ylang has strong sensual and euphoria-producing qualities, and the oil is heralded as an aphrodisiac. This essential oil is also renowned for its restorative powers and its relaxing effect on the nervous system. The oil is an antidepressant, and may be used therapeutically to treat stress, frustration, anger, and shock. It can have a balancing effect on blood pressure and distressed breathing patterns. Although it is used in many cosmetics for its fragrance, ylang ylang is also included in skin preparations for its balancing and toning effects.

Properties
Antiseptic • nervine • sedative • relaxing • soothing • antidepressant • balancing • aphrodisiac

The warm and lasting floral scent of ylang ylang blends well with bergamot, melissa, sandalwood and jasmine.

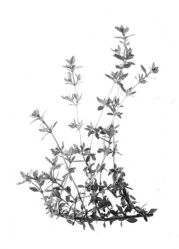

Using Essential Oils

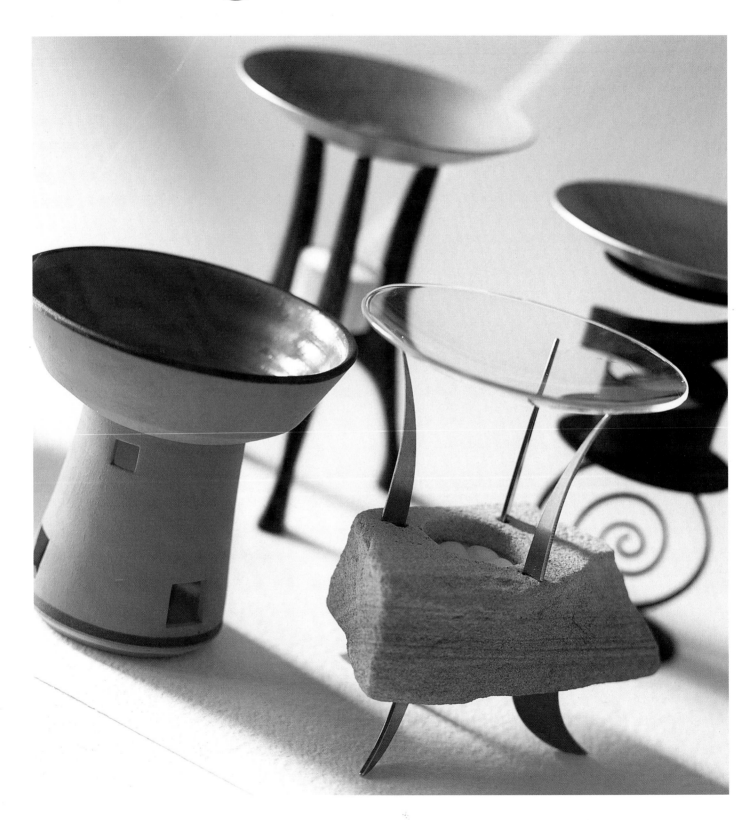

There are many ways to experience the benefits of essential oils. You may either breathe in the enticing aromas or absorb the diluted oils through the skin.

Direct application

Not usually recommended. Lavender and tea tree are the exceptions. Apply a dampened cotton swab or sterile cotton gauze cloth, dipped in a drop of oil, to the affected spot.

Massage oils

Add your chosen essential oils to base carrier oils for massage and beauty treatments. Measure 2 oz (50 ml) base carrier oil (see page 26) into a glass bowl or bottle, add 10–25 drops essential oils, and blend. Do not make up more than about a week's worth of blended oils. Store your massage blend in a well-sealed dark glass bottle in a cool dark place, and shake the bottle well before each use.

For massage, the usual proportion is about 2–3 drops essential oils to 1 teaspoon (5 ml) carrier oil. You need only about a spoonful for each massage. Where a stronger blend is indicated for healing, use about 15 drops in 1 oz (30 ml).

Baths

Fill the bathtub with hand-hot water and then add the essential oils. Disperse the oils well before getting in. Use about 6–12 drops of essential oil for each bath. Alternatively, rub on some blended massage oil before getting into the bathtub.

IMPORTANT

The extraction of essential oils is an extremely intensive process and can result in a rather expensive product. However, a true oil is very concentrated and requires only a tiny amount to work its wonders. Be sure to buy your oils from a reliable, informed supplier who can advise you if the oil has been blended. Although some essential oils, such as lavender, are safe even for the beginner to use, others are very strong and can be toxic if used undiluted.

Oils should be used under the guidance of a qualified herbalist or aromatherapist. This is particularly important if you suffer from high blood pressure, epilepsy, or a neural disorder, as some essential oils can aggravate these conditions. Similarly, certain oils should be avoided during pregnancy as they can trigger menstruation or miscarriage. If you have sensitive skin or suffer from allergies, consult an aromatherapist before using any essential oil. If in doubt, do a patch test first.

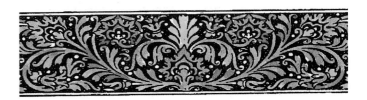

Footbaths

Add 4–8 drops essential oil to a bowl of warm to hot water. Soak for about 15 minutes to refresh the feet.

Sitz baths

Also called hip baths, these are a good method for localized healing. Fill a large plastic bowl with hot or cool to tepid water, depending on the treatment required. Add 6–8 drops essential oil and agitate the mixture before immersing the affected area.

Showers

Sprinkle 2-3 drops essential oil onto a damp cloth and rub over the body while under the shower.

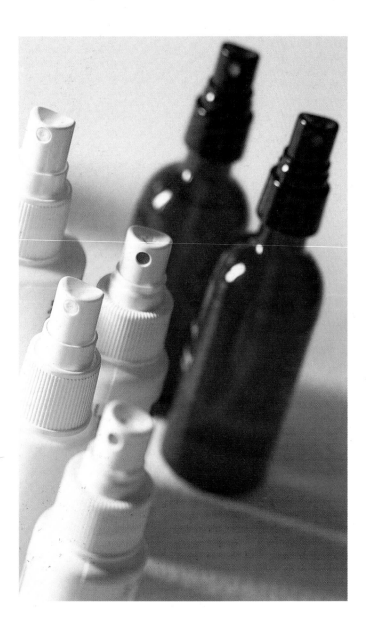

Compresses

Fill a bowl with hot or cold water and add 3–12 drops essential oils. Agitate well to disperse the oils. Place a cotton cloth, washcloth or towel on top of the water; squeeze out and apply to the area to be treated. Use hot compresses for arthritis, neuralgia, muscle ache, back pain, menstrual cramps, and skin inflammation. Use cold compresses for headaches, bruises, eye aches, and tension. For cramps, colic, swelling, sprains, and bruises, hot or cold compresses may be used. Leave on for about 20 minutes or until the compress reaches body temperature.

Inhalation

Use to hydrate, cleanse and stimulate the skin, and for mental fatigue, sinus problems, congestion, and colds. Fill a glass bowl with very hot, near-boiling water and add 4-10 drops of your chosen essential oils. Place a towel over the head and breathe deeply.

Another method of inhalation is to sprinkle a drop of essential oil onto a tissue or handkerchief.

Atomizers

These are also called sprays or spritzers. Use glass, not plastic, atomizers. Fill them with distilled, purified, spring, or mineral water. If bottled water is not available, use cooled boiled water. Add 3-6 drops of essential oil to each 1 oz (30 ml) of water. This should be enough for a day's immediate use. Refill as required. Use to fragrance a room or refresh your face.

Vaporizers

Also called fragrancers, burners, aroma lamps, and diffusers, these containers (usually ceramic) have a bowl at the top and an opening for a candle at the bottom. Fill the bowl with hot water and add the essential oils. The candle keeps the water heated, releasing the fragrance into the atmosphere. Use 5–15 drops of essential oil. Take care not to let the water evaporate completely, as the oils will leave a sticky residue in the bowl.

Light bulb rings

Pour the essential oil into these hollow rings. Then slip a ring over a light bulb and switch on the lights, so that the room will be filled with fragrance once the bulb heats up.

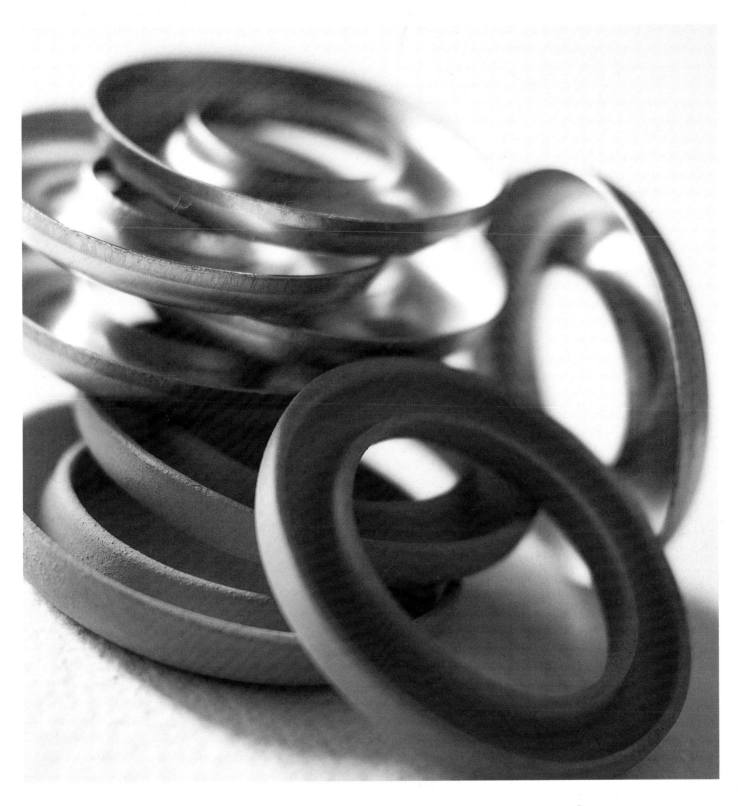

*Because essential oils are highly concentrated,
it is not usually advisable to apply them directly to your skin or
to ingest them, unless a skilled therapist suggests this.*

Blending and Storing Oils

For the greatest effect,
co-ordinate the oils you use daily
in massage blends,
perfumes, bath blends,
and your surroundings.
Don't combine too many oils,
as they may clash and be
overpowering.
A blend of four would be
the most complex
combination you should try.

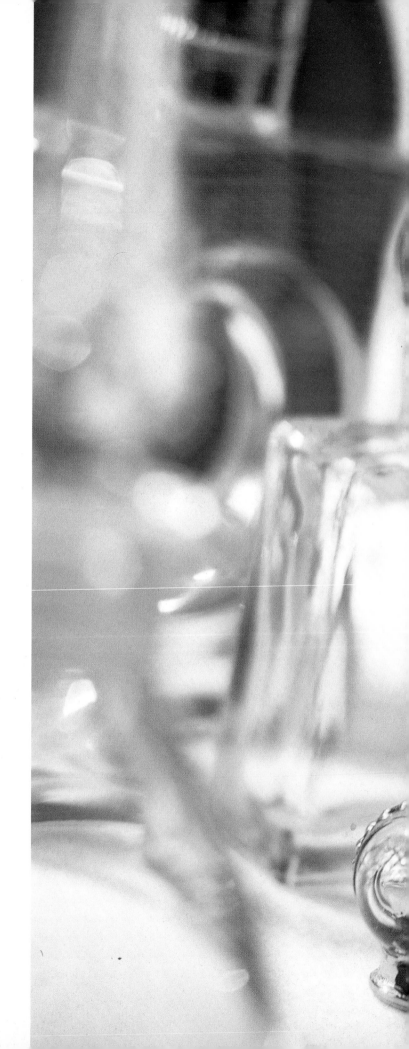

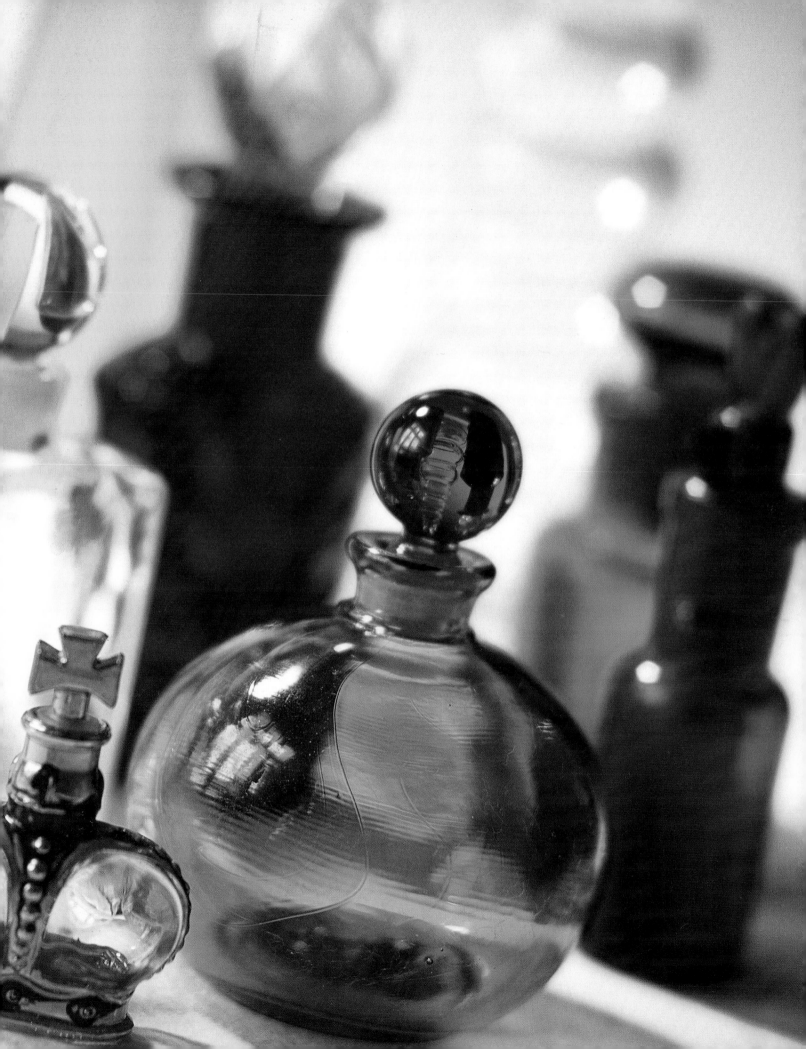

*B*ecause essential oils are very highly concentrated, they are best diluted to enhance the penetration of their active elements. For massage, for example, the concentrated oil should be added to a much greater quantity of another oil, known as a "carrier" or "base" oil.

Blending

A base carrier oil should have a neutral aroma and be easily absorbed. Use only 100% pure unrefined cold pressed vegetable, nut, or seed oils, not mineral oils. Sweet almond, apricot kernel, grapeseed, and peach kernel oil are all popular choices.

Base carrier blends for face and body

The proportion of essential oil to base carrier oil or water is the most important measurement to remember when making up a blend. Just because a little essential oil is beneficial, it does not mean that a large amount will work better. Use only tiny amounts: see the recommended proportions of essential oils to base carrier oils (see page 21), and use less for children or if you are pregnant.

Base carrier oils

Grapeseed
This clear, fine oil has no smell and is an excellent base carrier oil for massage.

Hazelnut
A good penetrative oil that is slightly astringent. This makes it a good choice for oily skins.

Jojoba
This is not an oil but a liquid wax, so it has the benefit of not turning rancid. Non-greasy and highly penetrative, it softens the skin and hair. Use 100% or add to other base oils.

Peach or apricot kernel oil
Good for mature, sensitive, or dry skin, this finely textured oil is recommended for facial use as it is rich in vitamins and great for cell regeneration.

Safflower
Good for all skin types.

Sunflower
Good for all skin types.

Sweet almond
Highly recommended, this is an excellent general-purpose base carrier oil that is neutral, non-allergenic, and good for all skin types.

Additions to base carrier oils

The following oils are used as additions to a base carrier oil, usually making up 10% of the total blend.

Avocado
This is a rich and heavy oil that is rarely used on its own, although it is very nourishing and therefore good for dry skin conditions. Add to base carrier oils to help penetration.

Evening primrose
This oil is also good for dry skin conditions and can make up 10% in a blend with other base carrier oils.

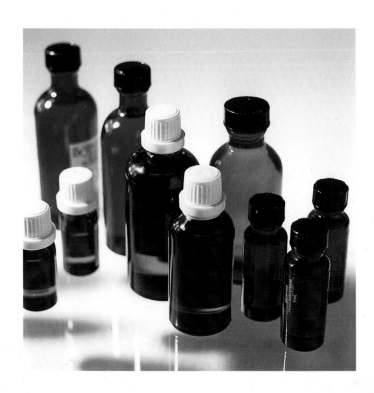

Olive

This is a good basic oil, but it has a strong aroma of its own so it is best used with other base carrier oils.

Vitamin E

Mix with base carrier oils such as sweet almond or jojoba to aid penetration of the skin. Good for facial use and for stretch marks.

Wheatgerm

Too rich and heavy to use on its own, this nourishing oil is good for mature skin and dry skin conditions. It is also an anti-oxidant, so add as 10% of a total blend to prevent oxidization and rancidity, and to provide vitamin E.

Storage

A few drops of your selected essential oil in 3 tablespoons base carrier oil should be sufficient for a massage. As a rough guide, you should not make up more than a week's worth of oil at one time as the fragrance spoils after a short while. Commercially purchased blends and lotions, however, usually contain some kind of anti-oxidant and so last longer.

Adding wheatgerm oil or vitamin E to your mixture can help to prevent it turning rancid. Keep your massage oil in dark glass bottles as these are best for reducing the deterioration of essential oils, and store in a cool dark place.

If blending oils with water in an atomizer, it is always preferable to make up your mixture daily.

CONVERSIONS

1 ml	*20 drops*	
5 ml	*1 teaspoon*	
10 ml	*2 teaspoons*	
20 ml	*1 tablespoon*	
1 oz 25–30 ml	*6 teaspoons*	
2 oz 50–60 ml	*2½ tablespoons*	
3 oz 90–100 ml	*5 tablespoons*	

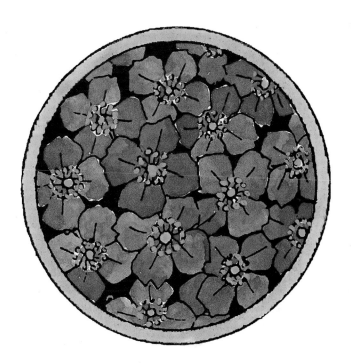

Oil classifications

Top note oils

Generally, the top note oils are the fastest acting and quickest to evaporate, lasting 3–24 hours. They tend to be the most stimulating and uplifting oils:
basil, bergamot, clary sage, eucalyptus, lemon, orange, peppermint, rosewood, sage, tea tree

Middle note oils

The middle note oils are moderately volatile, lasting 2–3 days, and affect the metabolism and body functions:
chamomile, cypress, geranium, juniper, lavender, marjoram, pine, rosemary, thyme

Base note oils

The base note oils are slower to evaporate, lasting up to 1 week, and are the most sedating and relaxing oils:
cedarwood, frankincense, jasmine, myrrh, neroli, patchouli, rose, sandalwood, ylang ylang

The Aromatherapy Massage

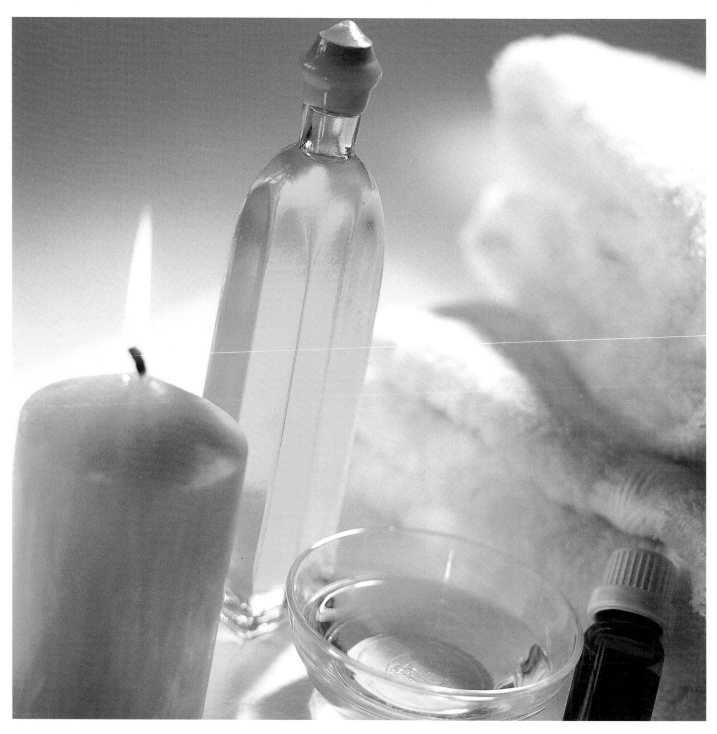

*A*romatherapy massage may be relaxing, invigorating or uplifting, depending on the oil chosen. Any massage technique can be used in conjunction with aromatherapy but the most common is the more gentle and relaxing form of Swedish massage. Others include acupressure, lymphatic drainage, and facial massage. The benefits are innumerable and involve emotional, mental, and physical effects, both curative and restorative. This is not only from the therapeutic effects of the oils, but also from the massage itself.

The touch of massage can convey reassurance, calm, relaxation, warmth, and understanding. On a physical level, it will:

- improve your circulation and your body's healing process,
- relax your nervous system,
- sooth tense muscles,
- remove toxins from your body.

A massage with a loved one can be a sensual experience, where you learn to trust and to give.

In this chapter, you will be taken step-by-step through a massage you can follow at home. There are very few rules, and a massage is a very enjoyable thing to give or to receive.

Creating the environment

- Ensure you have privacy and won't be interrupted.
- Play soft, soothing music if you find it helps you to relax.
- Keep the lighting soft and subtle; candlelight is ideal, and an eye patch is handy when lying on the back.
- The room should be comfortably warm and free of drafts.
- A vaporizer can be used — however, the massage oils will provide enough fragrance.

Accessories

Unless you have a professional massage table, the best place to massage at home is on the floor on a thin foam mat or folded blankets covered by a sheet. A thick soft mattress or futon is *not* recommended as it will counteract much of the pressure applied by the masseuse.

You will also need to have on hand two pillows, several towels (bath and hand size), a blanket for covering the body, and possibly a hot water bottle for the feet.

For information on massage oils, see page 21.

Giving a massage

You should be relaxed and comfortable as any tension will be communicated to your partner.

Clean your hands and stretch them to increase sensitivity and flexibility. Wear loose clothing. Watch your posture. If you are not comfortable in any position, move to one where you are. Remember to use the weight of your body when applying any pressure to lessen strain on yourself.

A WARNING

It may not be appropriate to be massaged if you have any of the following conditions:

- suffered a recent trauma — fractured bones, whiplash, sprains, etc.
- an acute inflammatory condition — signs include redness, swelling, pain, or loss of function
- recent damage to ligaments, tendons, or muscles
- skin problems, burns, sores, etc
- thrombosis
- tumour or cancers
- recent surgery

Care should be taken with the following conditions. Check with a doctor or therapist:

- high blood pressure or a heart condition
- pregnancy
- loose joints and joint replacements
- osteoporosis or brittle bones
- multiple sclerosis
- diabetes
- varicose veins

The basic massage movements

In Swedish massage — which forms the basis of most aromatherapy massage — there are a number of basic techniques which are very useful to learn, as they are frequently repeated throughout the massage.

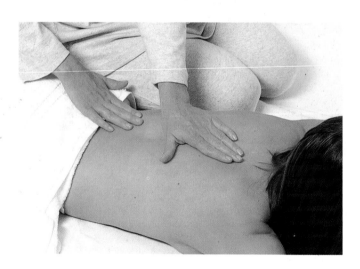

Stroking

Stroking is very important as it establishes the first contact with the patient. It will also help you locate areas of muscle tightness or pain. Long, gentle strokes are used to spread oil over the area being massaged. Both hands may stroke at one time, or alternate. On the legs or hands, stroking is usually in the direction of the feet or hands. Stroking should always be relaxing, soothing and comforting — use a light touch.

Effleurage

Effleurage warms the area being massaged and promotes circulation. It also has a relaxing effect on tight, tense muscles.

Effleurage is generally a long, even stroke applied with firm pressure. It is a movement that has two parts.

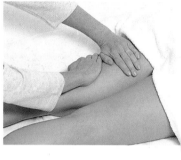

First, slide your hands forward. Generally, both hands work at the same time, either side by side with thumbs touching, or one below the other as illustrated in the first picture. When used on the back of your partner, you may move your hands in any direction, but on the limbs the movement should always be in the direction of the heart — this is the opposite to stroking.

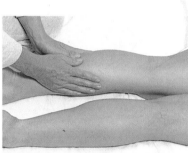

Second, after sliding hands forward, draw them back lightly in the opposite direction, as in the second picture.

Petrissage

Petrissage helps to relieve muscle fatigue and eliminate the buildup of toxins. It includes a range of movements, such as kneading, rolling, wringing and squeezing. While stroking and effleurage are long, gliding movements, petrissage concentrates more on a specific muscle areas to "soften them up" for deeper massage.

Kneading is just like kneading bread. Use each hand alternately to hold and squeeze flesh between your fingers.

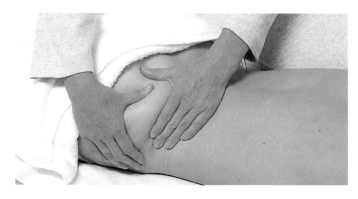

30

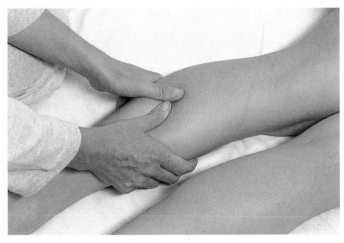

Frictions

Frictions work at a deeper level, concentrating on just a small section of the body at one time. This movement is designed to penetrate problem areas of tension buildup.

Generally the pads of the thumbs or fingers are used to create small circular movements. It is also possible to use the heel of the hand. Work slowly and carefully into the area — start gently and increase pressure as you feel the tissue relaxing beneath your fingers.

Percussion

If the aim of the massage is to quietly soothe your partner, percussion may be too vigorous. However, it can be a great stress reducer and very uplifting. If you do decide to use percussion movements, follow with flowing movements such as stroking. Make sure to keep your wrists loose.

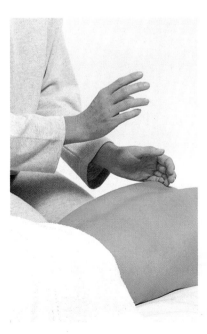

Flicking

Also known as hacking. In this movement the hands are relaxed, with palms facing one another. Use the little finger side of the hands and gently flick the surface of the skin with one hand and then the other. Keep the hands close together and try to form an even rhythm. The hands should be loose, bouncing easily off your partner's skin.

Plucking

This is a gentle and fairly rapid movement. Pick up the flesh between the thumb and fingers and then release, creating a plucking movement. Alternate the plucking from hand to hand to form a smooth rhythm.

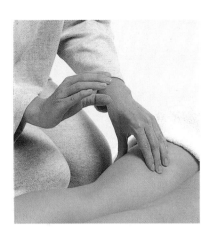

Cupping

Once again, keep wrists loose but form the hands into a cupped position, fingers touching lightly. The hands should be arched at the knuckles, forming a cavity. Each hand cups the surface of the skin alternately, keeping an even beat. This movement should create a loud, hollow sound.

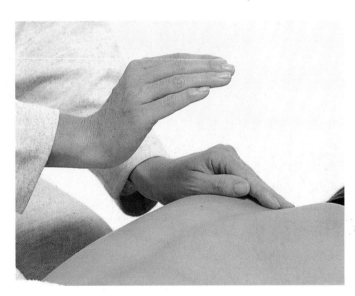

Pounding

Also known as pummelling, in this movement the hand is held in a loose fist. Use the little finger side of the fist, one hand after the other, to gently pound the muscle mass. Lift your fist off the skin straight away, creating a light, springy motion.

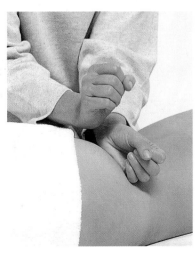

A full-body massage

After assessing your partner's condition, prepare a massage oil using 10-25 drops of your chosen essential oil or oils in 2 oz (50 ml) of base carrier oil

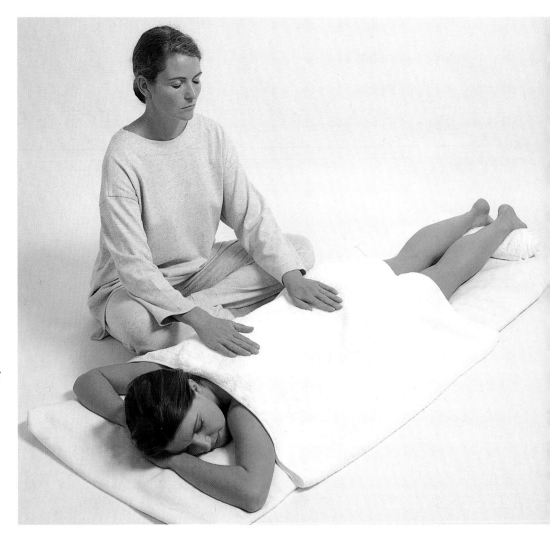

A few tips to keep in mind

• Try to maintain contact with your partner's body at all times during the massage; even when moving into a new position, try to keep one hand on the body.

• When massaging different parts of the body, keep the rest of the body covered with a large towel or blanket. This will keep your partner warm — this warmth will not only be soothing but shall also assist the therapeutic benefits of the massage and increase the absorption of oils used.

• Try not to talk too much throughout the massage as it will interrupt the process but do encourage your partner to let you know if there is any discomfort or a particular need.

• Always ensure your hands are warm before placing them anywhere near your partner — rub briskly together if they are at all cold.

A full body massage can be performed in any order. It is common to begin with the back or back of the legs, progressing to the front of legs, arms, abdomen, chest and finishing with the neck and face. However, this can be varied depending on preference.

Connecting

The most important parts of a massage are the beginning and the end. The initial touch will set the mood of the massage for both of you. Once your partner is comfortable and covered by a blanket or towel, gently place your hands on their body — one hand on the nape of the neck and the other on the small of the back, for example. Breathe slowly and deeply, close your eyes and let the energy flow between you. Very softly rock your partner's body from side to side. Focus in this position for several minutes before allowing your hands to lift from the body. Now you are ready to fold back the covering and begin massaging.

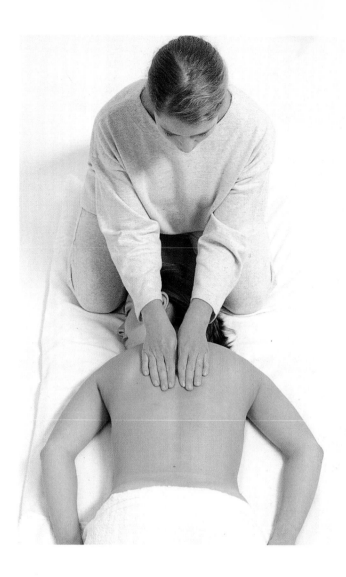

3. Moving on to the shoulders, knead the upper shoulder muscles. Gently squeeze and release around the whole shoulder area.

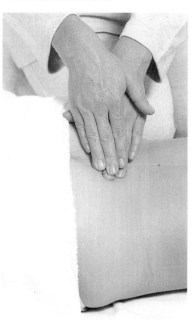

4. Move to one side of your partner, kneeling near their ribs. You will be massaging the side of the back opposite you. Place both hands on the buttock area, one hand on top of the other. Circle with the hands in wide, sweeping movements from the buttocks towards the head, covering the entire side up to the shoulders. Return, running your fingers lightly down the spine.

5. Knead the buttock area on the side opposite you, using squeezing and releasing movements.

6. Work a little deeper with frictions over the buttocks and base of spine. Use the pads of fingers to locate and work tight muscle areas.

7. Move to the other side of your partner and repeat movements 4 to 6.

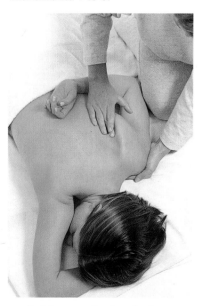

8. Kneel near the shoulder of your partner. It may be easiest if you lift your partner's arm and place their forearm on their lower back as shown. Slide your hand under their shoulder for support. Use your fingertips and the circular friction movement to massage the shoulder blade. Change sides and repeat.

9. Move to the head of your partner, and gently stroke from base of spine to neck. Cover the back with a towel and pat or rock gently.

The Back

Your partner should be lying face down with the head turned to one side — changing the direction of the head from time to time will help prevent a stiff neck. Position the arms where they are comfortable. A pillow under the ankles will add extra comfort and support.

1. Kneel near the head of your partner and apply a light coating of oil with long gentle stroking movements over the entire back and shoulders.

Using the effleurage stroke, glide your hands down each side of the spine then slide them back up the side of the body. Let your body lean into each movement as you work down the body and then back up. Repeat several times.

2. Work the muscle which runs each side of the spine. Using the friction movement, move your thumbs in circles from the top of the spine to the base — then return up the sides of body.

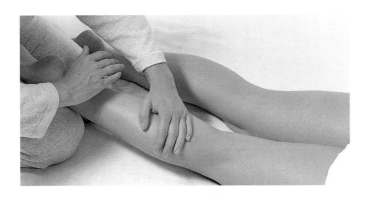

The legs

Uncover one leg, keeping the remainder of the body covered and warm. Try placing a pillow under the shin as it relieves pressure from the lower back.

1. Kneeling near the foot of your partner, apply oil with gentle stroking movements covering the entire leg, from thigh to ankle.

2. Using the effleurage movement, firmly glide both hands up the middle of the leg from ankle to the top of thigh. Return very gently down the sides of the leg to the ankle.

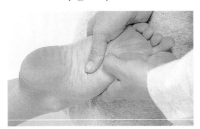

3. Kneel or sit cross-legged near your partner's toes and cradle the foot in one hand. Stroke the foot firmly with the other hand.

4. Rest the foot on your knee or in your lap and use your thumb in the friction movement to massage in small circles over the entire sole.

5. Now work on the calf of the leg — you may find it comfortable to place your partner's leg on your knee. The movement is a firm effleurage stroke, using only one hand at a time. Cupping your hands, stroke up the calf muscle with one hand — as it reaches the top of the calf, the other hand begins with the same movement from the ankle to form a rhythmic, flowing motion.

6. Having relaxed the area, now work more deeply into the muscle mass using circular thumb frictions. It is best to work up the calf, stroking upwards and outwards with the thumbs. Begin gently, increasing pressure gradually — many people are very sensitive in this area.

7. Move up to the thigh, repeating the same effleurage and friction movements.

8. You may now like to reposition yourself beside your partner's leg and try a series of kneading and percussion movements. Avoid the area around the back of the knee when using percussive movements.

9. Finish the leg massage with effleurage to the entire leg. End by softly drawing your fingers over the foot and off the edge of the toes.

10. Cover leg with a towel and pat entire area. Then repeat the entire process on the back of the other leg.

11. Ask your partner to roll over onto their back. Cover again with towels and place a pillow under the knees for support. Repeat the same process on the front of the legs but concentrate on the upper thigh. Remember there is no real muscle mass on the front of the lower legs so stroking and gentle kneading is all that is required.

The arm

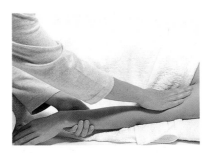

Cover the legs and reposition yourself so that you are kneeling beside your partner's arm. Apply oil with stroking movements to the whole arm.

1. Hold the arm softly at the wrist with one hand, while effleuraging with the other. Stroke from the lower arm to upper arm, glide around the shoulder and slide back down to the hand.

2. Concentrate the same movements to the forearm. Next try circular friction movements to the area, on the front and then the back.

3. Now work on the upper arm, first with effleurage then with friction movements.

4. Follow with effleurage to the entire arm.

5. Hold your partner's hand in yours and rub the palm with your thumb. Stroke the upper surface of the hand. Gently rotate the wrist; rotate the fingers and very softly pull them away from the hand.

6. Conclude the arm massage by gently stroking from shoulders to hands; on the final stroke let your hands glide lightly off your partner's. Cover the arm with a towel and pat gently.

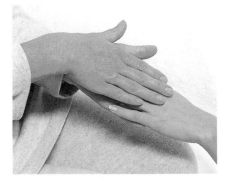

7. Repeat process on the other arm.

The abdomen and chest

1. Arrange towels so only the area from the rib cage to the pelvis is exposed.

2. Kneel on one side of your partner near the waist. Apply oil to the whole area with gentle, stroking movements. Effleurage up the middle of the abdomen, out over the lower ribs and down towards the waist. Pull back down to the lower abdomen, and repeat the whole movement.

3. Cover the area with a towel, and place both your hands on the abdomen, applying gentle pressure, before allowing the hands to lift from the area.

4. Follow with massage to the chest area. You can cover the breasts if you wish, leaving the upper chest area and shoulders exposed.

5. Kneel at the head of your partner and apply the oil by gliding hands down the middle of chest. Separate the hands, go around the breast area and return up the sides of body.

6. Knead the upper pectoral area — the fleshy area below the collarbone.

7. Using the pads of the fingers and light pressure only, work with friction movements over the breastbone.

8. Move to the side of your partner, and with the palms of your hands alternately stroke over the ribs opposite you, towards the middle of your partner's body. Repeat on the other side.

9. Finish by repeating the movements in step 5, then cover the area with a towel.

The neck

This is a very important area, as most of us store a lot of tension in the neck and upper shoulders.

1. Place a rolled towel under your partner's head. Turn the head to one side and gently stroke with your thumb from the base of the skull to the collarbone. While the head is in this position, knead the upper shoulder muscle. Turn the head to the other side, and repeat.

2. With the head facing straight up, place both your hands under the base of the neck, and using the pads of the fingers create circular movements up the neck to the base of the skull. The circles should be quite large.

3. Use small friction movements with the pads of the fingers along the base of the skull — work out to the ears and back. This area, where the head joins the neck, is often very tender.

4. Finish by stroking with both hands from shoulders to back of scalp.

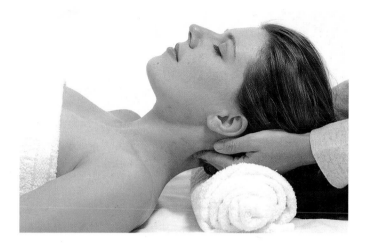

The face and scalp

It is very relaxing to conclude a massage with the face and scalp which will gently soothe away any remnants of tension and leave your partner in a state of blissful calm.

1. Sit at the head of your partner and begin with stroking the forehead.

2. Facial massage can be very intuitive. You may like to follow some of the suggestions outlined on page 53.

3. Don't forget to incorporate a scalp massage, using a "shampooing" motion over the entire area.

4. Finish by gently stroking over the forehead with the heels of the thumbs and the side of face with the fingers.

5. Finally, rub hands together till they are very warm, and hold just touching, and completely covering, your partner's face. Hold for several minutes, allowing your partner to drink in the warmth.

The closing touch

Now that you have completed your full body massage, make sure the whole of your partner's body is covered. Move to their side and place one hand on the forehead, the other on the abdomen. Close your eyes, and gently rock backwards and forwards — this is a very soothing, subtle movement. Remain in this position for some time, and then allow your hands to float off your partner's body.

The massage is now complete. You may like to cover your partner with an extra blanket, and suggest they rest before attempting to rise.

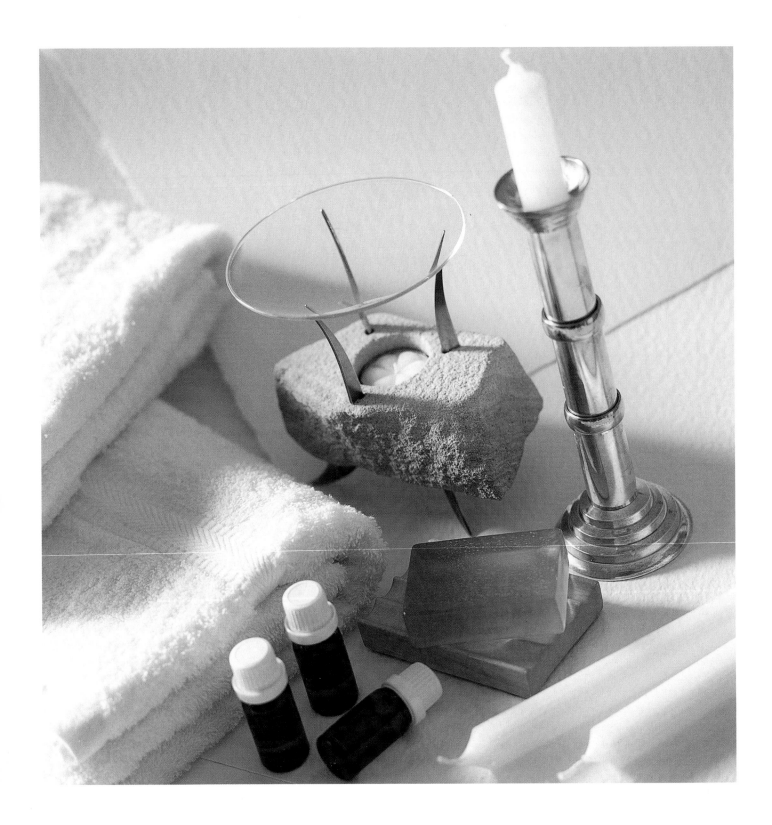

If you are looking for a bath that is relaxing, calming and balancing, experiment with these oils: bergamot, cedarwood, chamomile, clary sage, frankincense, geranium, lavender, marjoram, neroli, patchouli, rose.

The Aromabath

*Wait until
the bathtub is
almost full before adding
the oils, as they evaporate quickly.
Make sure they are well-dispersed
in the water so that there is no
irritation to your skin.*

Taking a bath is relaxing in itself, but if you add a few drops of essential oil the experience will be both sensual and therapeutic. Aromabaths can be detoxifying, relaxing, or reviving, depending on the oil or oils you choose. Sedating baths are wonderful just before bedtime, to dispel stress that may keep you awake. They are also a great way to relieve pain, boost the immune system and calm the body so that it can concentrate on recovery.

In the aromabath the therapeutic properties of the oils are dispersed in two ways: the heat of the water opens the pores and relaxes the muscles, aiding the absorption of the oils through the skin and into the circulatory system, and the steam from the bath enables the fragrance to be inhaled through the olfactory system.

Preparing a bath

To prepare an aromabath, simply add 4-12 drops of your selected oil(s) to a bathtub filled with warm water. The water should be "hand hot", that is, as hot as you can stand it, but not so hot that you will feel faint. Avoid very hot water if you are pregnant or have a heart condition, varicose veins, or broken capillaries. Stir the water well to ensure the oil is evenly dispersed, and then relax in the scented water. A 10–20 minute soak should have the desired effect.

If preferred, you can add the richness of a base carrier oil to the bathtub to nourish and soften your skin. Mix the essential oils with 1 tablespoon base carrier oil before adding to the bath water, or massage yourself with the oil before sinking into the bathtub. Sweet almond oil and jojoba oil work well in aromabaths.

Creating atmosphere

To really enjoy the simple indulgence of an aromabath, add to the effect with candlelight and soft music. Support your head on a bath pillow or a rolled-up towel, close your eyes, and inhale. Concentrate on your breathing, and empty your mind of worries. After 15–20 minutes, get out of the bathtub slowly and wrap yourself in a large, warm towel or robe. Sip a glass of water or try a soothing cup of chamomile tea if you want to relax further.

A refreshing bath

Aromabaths can pick you up as well as helping you to wind down. Keep the bath water tepid while you soak, then keep adding cool water to the bathtub to rinse. Or rinse under a cool shower. Rub yourself vigorously with a towel to dry off and splash your face with cold water.

Use invigorating and stimulating oils such as cypress, eucalyptus, fennel, geranium, juniper, lavender, lemon, lemongrass, peppermint, pine, rosemary, or thyme. Try a refreshing bath for a kick-start in the morning, after a long journey or before an evening out.

Oils for Health

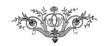

Essential oils have been used for centuries for healing. In recent years, this age-old knowledge has been backed up by scientific research. It has been proved that, among other medicinal qualities, essential oils have antiviral, antiseptic, antibacterial, antifungal and anti-inflammatory properties.

The therapeutic blends in this chapter are offered as natural tools to assist in the treatment of common health conditions. They will stimulate the healing of both mind and body.

The suggestions for treatment encompass the methods of using oils that are outlined in *Using Essential Oils* (page 20), and *Blending and Storing Oils* (page 24) should be consulted for information on blending. It is generally not advised to apply essential oils directly to the skin or to ingest them unless supervised by an aromatherapist.

Allergies

To reduce the symptoms of allergic reactions such as hay fever, mix 1 drop lavender oil in 1 teaspoon base carrier oil, and massage this mixture into your sinus area throughout the day. Carry the mixture around with you in a small bottle for easy access.

Arthritis

Try adding 3 drops lavender and 3 drops rosemary oil to a warm bath; the rosemary is for swelling and the lavender is for inflammation. If the joint is particularly painful, you can add 4 drops chamomile instead, as this oil is an effective analgesic. Or add 3 drops marjoram for extra effectiveness.

Asthma

Avoid steam inhalations, as these can aggravate the condition. Instead, try 2 drops peppermint oil on a handkerchief or tissue. Keep this with you and inhale it deeply throughout the day. The peppermint will help to clear your air passages.

Because asthma may be caused by a variety of factors, ongoing treatment may vary. If the asthma is triggered by an emotional condition, bergamot or chamomile may help, as they are antispasmodic and reduce depression. Lavender could help if the asthma is linked to a chest infection; try massaging the chest, neck, and throat with 10 drops essential oil blended in 3 teaspoons base carrier oil.

Bites and stings

Mix together 3 drops tea tree and 4 drops lavender oil with 3 teaspoons base carrier oil. Apply a little to the sting or bite every hour until the pain is relieved. An effective insect repellent can be made by adding 7 drops citronella essential oil to 3 teaspoons lanolin-free cream (not a vegetable oil-based cream); apply to exposed areas of skin. Or try burning a citronella candle.

Bladder infections

Taking an aromabath or using a sitz bath (see page 22) are effective ways of using essential oils to treat bladder infections such as cystitis, because the oil is applied directly to the affected area. Try 2 drops each eucalyptus, cedarwood, and sandalwood in a bathtub; make sure the oils are well dispersed before you get in.

Bronchitis

Try an inhalation of 3 drops each eucalyptus and lemon, added to a bowl of steaming water. If the steam irritates your breathing, it may be best to inhale the oil from a tissue. Alternatively, massage your chest and neck with a mix of 7 drops eucalyptus, 5 drops tea tree, and 3 drops lavender oil in 1 oz (30 ml) base carrier oil.

Bruises

Add 1 drop each of lavender and chamomile to a cold compress and apply to the bruised area; reapply as the compress warms. Alternatively, add 3 drops marjoram, 3 drops geranium and 1 drop chamomile oil to 1/2 teaspoon base carrier oil. Apply this mixture to the bruise immediately, and continue applying every 2 hours until it clears up. Be careful with this mixture on broken skin.

The recommendations in this book are useful home remedies but they are not meant to replace treatment by a medical practitioner. Before treating any health condition, always consult both your doctor and a qualified aromatherapist.

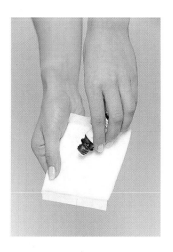

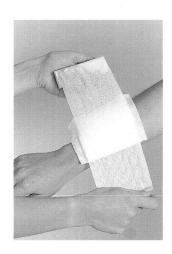

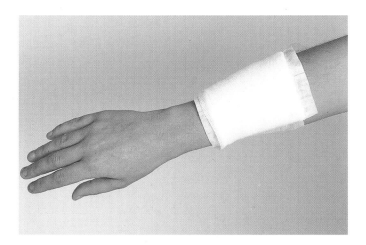

In a first-aid emergency,
lavender oil can be applied without dilution to a burn.
First, rinse the burn well under cool, running water for 5 to 20 minutes.
Next, add lavender oil to a clean gauze pad and
place lightly on the burn area.
Finally, gently wrap gauze bandage around the pad and
fasten to keep it in place.

Burns

For a severe burn you must seek medical advice, but for a minor burn lavender can really help. Lavender oil can be applied directly to the skin or mixed in with aloe vera gel.

It is very important that you first hold the burnt area under cool running water for at least 5 minutes, and up to 20 minutes if possible. Make up a blend of 7 drops lavender to 3 teaspoons aloe vera gel; mix well. Gently apply some of this blend to the burn, and cover with clean, sterile gauze. Every time you change the gauze, apply more lavender oil mixture. As the burn heals, you could also apply the lavender oil blend every morning and night.

For sunburn, dilute 5 drops lavender in 16 fl oz (500 ml) water (not oil). Spray on with an atomizer, or soak a cold cotton compress or handkerchief in the mixture to cool the burn. A tepid bath with 6 drops peppermint and 4 drops lavender may also help sooth and heal the skin.

Circulation problems

To improve your circulation if you have low blood pressure, try adding 4 drops rosemary to the bathtub, making sure the oil is well dispersed.

Colds and flu

The two most common methods for treating colds are inhalations and aromabaths. The steam from aromabaths may also help your breathing. Baths have the added benefit of relaxing the body and giving it a chance to heal. If you have trouble sleeping because of painful sinuses, a bath with 2 drops lavender and 2 drops marjoram should help.

During the day, place 2 drops rosemary and 1 drop peppermint in a vaporizer with some water, to fight the bacteria in the air and clear your sinuses. Avoid these oils at night as they are stimulants and may keep you awake.

For chest infection, massage the chest with a mix of 10 drops tea tree oil in 1 oz (30 ml) base carrier oil.

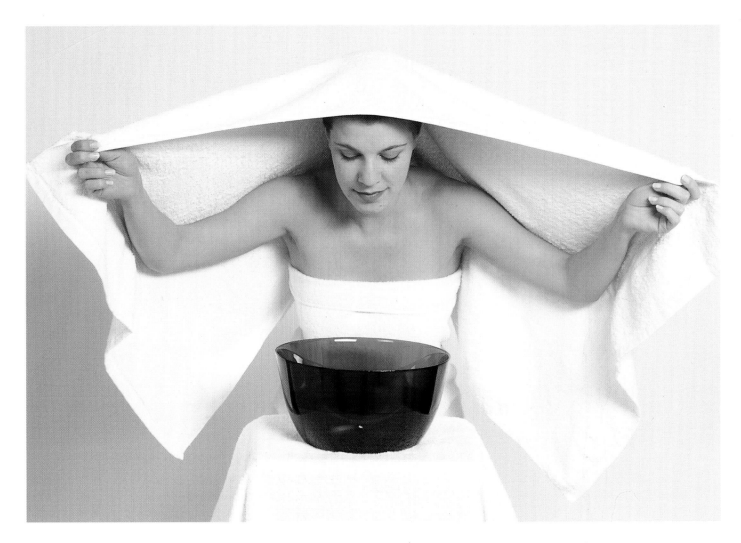

For a cough, use a massage blend of 5 drops eucalyptus, 4 drops peppermint, 3 drops basil, and 3 drops pine oil in 1 oz (30 ml) base carrier oil.

If you have laryngitis, massage your throat and chest with a massage blend of 5 drops lavender, 4 drops chamomile, and 4 drops tea tree oil in 1 oz (30 ml) base carrier oil.

For tonsillitis, sit for as long as you can in a bathtub containing 2 drops eucalyptus and 1 drop peppermint oil, making sure the oil is properly dispersed. For throat infections, gargle with 1 drop bergamot or tea tree oil added to a glass of water.

Constipation

Add 2 drops marjoram and 2 drops rosemary oil to 2 teaspoons base carrier oil. Massage this into your stomach lightly in a clockwise direction for 5 minutes. Or you could get someone else to do it for you. Alternatively, add 5 drops each fennel and rosemary to your bath water.

Inhalations can soothe inflamed mucous membranes and clear the sinuses. Try 2 drops eucalyptus and 2 drops tea tree oil in a bowl of steaming water for colds or flu. Inhalations can also be useful for other respiratory ailments, although sometimes the steam may irritate the lungs. The same technique of "tenting" the head is also used for facial steaming.

Cramps

Aromabaths are also good for relaxing the body, and therefore work in the prevention and relief of cramps. A massage will assist circulation, and can ease cramping muscles. Use a blend of 5 drops each marjoram and basil in your bath water, or add 1 drop each to $1/2$ teaspoon base carrier oil for massage. Try also lavender and geranium.

*Be careful about using
the same oils for weeks on end,
because you can get a
build-up in your body of toxic
constituents and
this can be dangerous.*

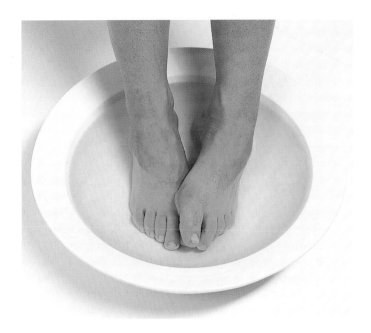

A warm footbath is a treat for tired,
aching feet. Afterwards, sit with
your feet elevated for a few
minutes to give them a further rest
and assist circulation.

Depression

Depression can take several forms, and there are oils suited to all the varying types. There are sedative oils that help depression when it is accompanied by insomnia and restlessness, and there are oils that lift the mood without sedating — these are good for depression that causes fatigue and lethargy. Often it is best for you to decide which oil is appropriate — just trust your instincts.

Touch is also important when you are depressed. Often the feel of someone's hands on your body will make you feel more secure. If you need to be uplifted and also soothed, ask someone to give you a massage using a mixture of 2 drops each chamomile, geranium, and lavender oil in 3 teaspoons base carrier oil. Or use these oils in a comforting bath.

Diarrhea

Oils that have a soothing effect on the intestinal lining and lessen diarrhea include chamomile, lavender, neroli, and peppermint. You can add them to baths, include them in a massage oil, or burn them in a vaporizer in your room. Try inhaling neroli from a tissue before a nerve-racking event to calm yourself and prevent nervous diarrhea.

Fatigue

Take a bath with 2 drops rosemary and 2 drops basil oil, making sure the oils are well dispersed in the bathtub. You can also sprinkle 2 drops rosemary oil onto a tissue and inhale it throughout the day. Put the tissue inside your shirt and the warmth will help to further release the aroma. Avoid these oils before bedtime as they are stimulating.

Feet

Take a warm footbath containing 4 drops lavender and 2 drops marjoram oil. The marjoram will relieve pain and the lavender will soothe. You may like to massage your feet or have them massaged by a friend while you take the footbath.

If your feet are swollen, 3 drops each bergamot and chamomile oil may help.

For smelly feet, try adding 6 drops sage oil to a footbath.

A refreshing footbath can be made with 3 drops each peppermint and lemon oil.

Fluid retention

These essential oils have diuretic qualities to help relieve fluid retention: juniper, lavender, and rosemary.

If your fluid retention is due to premenstrual swelling, make up a warm compress using 3 drops each juniper and lavender and 2 drops rosemary. Place the compress over your abdomen and breasts for 10 minutes for a few nights before your period.

Hangover

To ease the headache, try applying a cold compress with 4 drops geranium and 1 drop lemon or lavender to the temples. For symptoms like nausea, see the relevant entries.

Headaches

The two oils most effective for headache relief are lavender and peppermint. They clear the head and relieve pain, and are far safer than the ubiquitous aspirin.

Make a cold compress from a damp cotton pad, adding 2 drops each lavender and peppermint oil. Apply this to the forehead, the temples, or the back of the head, wherever the headache is.

If your headache is due to sinusitis, make up a steam inhalation containing 2 drops each eucalyptus, lavender, and rosemary oil.

Indigestion

Oils that have a calming effect on the stomach and help digestion include chamomile, lavender, peppermint, and marjoram.

Ask someone to give you a gentle massage on your stomach and abdominal area with a mixture of 2 drops each chamomile and lavender in 3 teaspoons base carrier oil. The massage should be given in a clockwise direction and only last a few minutes (see page 28 for massage details).

Five to 10 drops lavender in a vaporizer can help to reduce heartburn.

Menopause

If you are experiencing a hot flush, sprinkle 2 drops peppermint on a tissue and inhale until you feel cooler.

Take a relaxing bath in warm water into which 2 drops each geranium and rose have been added.

An aromatherapy travel kit

If you take the following selection of essential oils with you when you travel, you should be prepared for most common ailments and injuries.

Chamomile
diarrhea, exhaustion, insomnia

Eucalyptus
*colds, cramps, cuts, fever,
heat exhaustion*

Geranium
*blisters, dehydrated skin,
exhaustion, heat cramps*

Lavender
*burns, cuts, dehydrated skin,
diarrhea, fever, headaches,
heat exhaustion, insects,
insomnia, skin infections, sprains*

Peppermint
*diarrhea, exhaustion, fever,
headaches, indigestion, insects,
nausea, toothache*

Tea tree
colds, skin infections, thrush

Nausea

Inhalations are the most effective and convenient ways of treating nausea (a few drops of oil sprinkled on a tissue work well), but you can also have a gentle abdominal massage or take a soothing bath with the suggested oils.

If your nausea is associated with emotional problems, the best oils to use are lavender and sandalwood.

If food has upset your stomach or you have travel sickness (or if wish to prevent either ailment), peppermint oil is recommended.

Nosebleeds

Soak a piece of absorbent cotton in cold water that contains 1 drop lemon oil. Insert this into your bleeding nostril and leave in until the bleeding has slowed.

Pain

There are many aromatherapy oils that help to reduce pain, whether muscular or internal. These include bergamot, chamomile, lavender, marjoram, and rosemary.

Your skin can absorb these oils via an aromabath, a body massage, steam inhalation, tissue inhalation, or a vaporizer.

For muscular pain, try a hot compress of 2 drops chamomile, 2 drops rosemary, and 1 drop sandalwood oil, or a massage with a blend of 5 drops juniper, 4 drops lavender, and 4 drops rosemary oil in 1 oz (30 ml) base carrier oil. A warm bath containing 2 drops rosemary and 2 drops lavender oil can work wonders.

Panic attacks

Sprinkle 2 drops lavender oil onto a tissue and inhale deeply and slowly. Lavender calms the mind and body, and the act of deep breathing brings the body into a calmer state. A small bottle of lavender oil is easily portable and great to have on hand if you are expecting a stressful time.

42

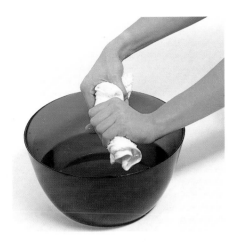

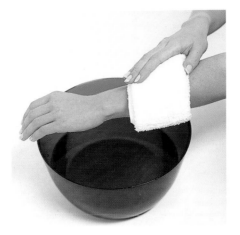

Make a compress by adding a few drops of your chosen essential oil to a bowl of water, mixing it well. Saturate a clean cloth in the water, wring out excess and apply to the part of your body requiring treatment. Reapply when it reaches body temperature.

Period pain

Apply a warm compress containing 2 drops each chamomile, clary sage, and marjoram oil to your back and lower abdomen. Or try taking a bath with 4 drops clary sage, 3 drops geranium, and 3 drops rose oil.

Premenstrual tension

For mood swings, depression and irritability, use clary sage, bergamot, jasmine, or rose oil. Some of the other essentials oils that can balance the emotions include chamomile, geranium, lavender, and sandalwood. To get the best results, you can start using these oils in baths and massage as much as 10 days before your period begins.

Skin problems

If you have eczema, combine 4 drops each chamomile, juniper, and geranium oil with 5 teaspoons base carrier oil. Apply a portion of this mixture every morning and night to the affected areas until the condition clears.

For other skin rashes, try taking a warm (not hot) bath with 4 drops each chamomile and lavender oil. Or add 2 drops of each to a cool compress.

Chapped skin will benefit from being steamed once a week over a basin of very hot water to which 2 drops geranium oil have been added. Then massage in a mixture of 2 drops chamomile, 1 drop lavender, and 1 drop patchouli oil to 2 teaspoons carrier base oil.

Thrush

Add 2 drops each myrrh and tea tree oil to your bath water, making sure the oil is well dispersed. As you sit in the bathtub, swish the water toward you to ensure contact. Or use a sitz bath. These oils will reduce infection and soothe the itching and soreness of exposed areas.

Toothache

Add a drop of clove oil to a moistened cotton swab or cotton bud and apply to affected area.

Varicose veins

Apply the following mixture to the affected areas every morning: 3 drops cypress, 3 drops sandalwood, and 1 drop peppermint oil to 5 teaspoons base carrier oil. Use the palms of your hands to apply the oil and work up your legs toward your heart rather than down. Don't actually massage the veins themselves, but work around them.

Viral infections

Some of the essential oils used for treating viral infections include bergamot, eucalyptus, juniper, lavender, and tea tree. You should never allow anyone to massage you if you have a high fever, as the massage may aggravate the fever. Rather, take a bath in tepid water for at least 15 minutes with 3 drops of any of the above oils.

Warts

Try a mixture of 7 drops lemon oil in 3 teaspoons base carrier oil. Apply to the wart before covering with sticking plaster. Do this every day until the wart becomes smaller and drops off.

Wounds

Dilute any of the following on absorbent cotton, and apply to the wound: bergamot, eucalyptus, geranium, lemon, or rose oil. Lavender and tea tree oil can also be applied directly, without dilution, and will keep the area free of bacteria.

Oils for Pregnancy

If you are pregnant,
use only low doses of
essential oils.
A basic massage bl[...]
of 3 drops essential [...]
to 2-3 teaspoons bas[...]
carrier oil is
recommended.

- relieving pain
- fatigue

Pregnancy is a time of physical and emotional change, and essential oils can help you cope with the demands that are being made on you. Essential oil baths and massages are great at relieving pain and fatigue during pregnancy and help with stress relief. It is best to consult a professional aromatherapist during pregnancy so as to avoid any possible complications, and to make the most of this therapy.

Oils for aromabaths
Refreshing: bergamot, lemon, orange, neroli
Soothing: neroli, ylang ylang
Relaxing: geranium, lavender

Oils for massage
Abdomen: lavender, neroli
Legs and feet: geranium, lavender
Lower back: bergamot, geranium, sandalwood
Relaxation: frankincense, neroli, sandalwood

Although aromatherapy can be a great help if you are pregnant, there are many oils you should avoid because they can induce menstruation and deplete fluid in the foetal sac. It is best to avoid all essential oils for the first three months of pregnancy, or if you have a history of miscarriage.

Avoid throughout your whole pregnancy
angelica, anise, arnica, basil, birch, camphor, caraway, carrot, cedarwood, cinnamon, clary sage, clove, cypress, fennel, hyssop, jasmine, juniper, marjoram, mint, myrrh, nutmeg, oregano, pennyroyal, peppermint, rose, rosemary, sage, sassafras, savoury, sweet fennel, thyme, true melissa and wintergreen

Avoid in the first 3 months
(later they will be quite safe):
chamomile, frankincense, geranium, lavender, mandarin

Stretch marks

Regular massage from the fifth month of pregnancy will keep skin supple and can help prevent stretch marks. Try a blend of 10 drops lavender and 5 drops neroli in 2 oz (50 ml) of base carrier oil. Add Vitamin E or wheatgerm oil (to make up 10% of the total blend) for added skin nourishment. Even unperfumed oil (for example, almond) will make a difference to the elasticity of your skin.

For the birthing room

During the lead-up to the birth, essential oils can be used in massage blends and hot compresses for pain relief. Cool compresses wiped on the forehead and face between contractions will cool and relax you. Add your chosen essential oils to a bowl of hot water or in a vaporizer, to release soothing fragrances into the room.

Clary sage is effective for strengthening contractions.
Frankincense will help alleviate any fears you may have.
Lavender will be calming and relaxing.
Lemon and tea tree will freshen and disinfect the room.

For new mothers

Nursing your baby

Try 2 drops either fennel, lemongrass, or peppermint in a vaporizer to promote breast milk. Or massage with a mix of 1 drop of fennel, geranium, or clary sage in 1 teaspoon base carrier oil; wash off thoroughly before feeding. Fennel tea and peppermint tea are also recommended.

Sore breasts

Massage your breasts when they feel sore or after each feeding session, using a base carrier oil containing only a very low dose of essential oil (chamomile, geranium, lavender, peppermint, or rose). Massage from the outer edge of your breast toward your nipple — don't forget your underarm area. Avoid the nipple and remove all traces of oil before the next feed.

You can also use warm compresses before nursing your baby, and cold compresses after the feed.

Postnatal depression

Changing hormone levels mean that nearly half of all new mothers experience post-baby blues. Add a blend from the following oils to your bath or use in a massage to lift your spirits and give yourself some time to relax: bergamot, clary sage, frankincense, geranium, jasmine, lavender, lemon, neroli, orange, patchouli, rose, sandalwood, ylang ylang.

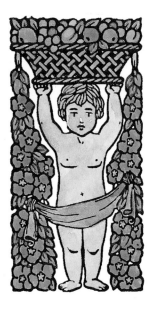

Aromatherapy for children

Children respond well to this gentle natural therapy. The fragrance is appealing, and a child's immune system can be effectively assisted with the healing oils. A few drops of soothing chamomile or lavender in a bath can calm over-tired, excitable, or irritable children, and help treat upset stomachs, rashes, and other childhood illnesses.

When bathing, changing, or feeding young children, it is easy to extend the contact into a gentle aromatherapy massage (see page 28). However, be very careful with the hot water needed for steam inhalations, and always keep vaporizers and the essential oils themselves well out of reach of children.

As a general rule, children over three years of age only require half the recommended adult dosage of an essential oil, and children under three years need only a quarter of the adult dose. For babies under eighteen months, use only 1 drop of oil in their bath.

Treating Stress

Stress may be the scourge of our modern way of life, but aromatherapy provides an effective antidote. You can use essential oils to help you relax and to stimulate you. They can calm you and refresh you, leaving you feeling balanced and grounded. The constituents of essential oils are closely related to human hormones, which makes them helpful in countering the effects of hormonal imbalance.

Aromatherapy works best as a preventative. You may be able to stop a small case of the "blues" turning into a deeper depression. Anxiety creates tension in the body and can trigger other stress-related symptoms and illnesses, such as headaches, backaches, or colds (see page 38 for details of how to treat these conditions).

If you want to reap the benefits of essential oils all day long when you are going through a stressful period, you can wear a suitable blend as a perfume (see page 59). Oils sprinkled on a tissue are a great method of instant assistance, making inhalation accessible whenever you feel the need for it. Atomizers too are portable, either as spritzers for your face or to spray a room. At the end of a tiring and frustrating day, an aromabath is soothing (see page 36). Ultimately, many people find the physical touch of a massage the most comforting of all — contact with another person can be supportive, stiffness can be gently worked out of muscles, and the whole process can be wonderfully indulgent.

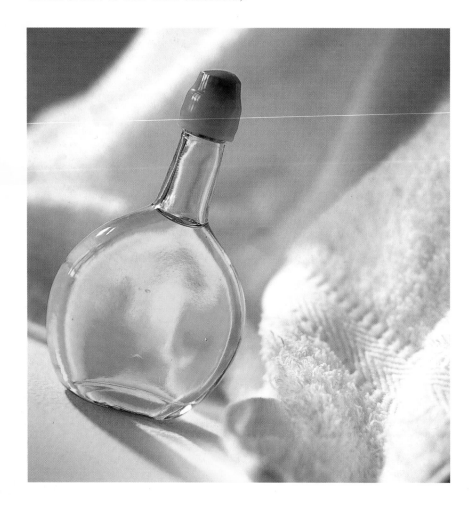

Lavender is one of the best treatments for insomnia or disturbed sleep. You can also try bergamot, marjoram, neroli, orange, or ylang ylang. Sprinkle a few drops of these oils on your bed linen, or use in a relaxing aromabath.

Essential oils
to counteract
negative
emotions

Anger
chamomile, rose, ylang ylang

Anxiety
basil, bergamot, geranium, lavender, neroli

Depression
geranium, lavender, bergamot,
clary sage, patchouli, ylang ylang

Fatigue
basil, bergamot, eucalyptus, juniper,
lemon, lemongrass,
orange, peppermint, rosemary, rosewood

Fear
frankincense, lavender, sandalwood

Forgetfulness
basil, rosemary

Grief
chamomile, rose

Irritability
lavender, neroli, rose, ylang ylang

Nervousness
basil, bergamot, cedarwood, geranium,
lavender, neroli

Resentfulness
rose

Stress
bergamot, lavender, neroli,
rose, sandalwood

Essential oils
to produce
positive
emotions

Balance
sandalwood

Comfort
lavender, rose, sandalwood

Concentration
basil, lemon, rosemary

Confidence
bergamot, cedarwood, frankincense,
jasmine, neroli, rose, sandalwood

Euphoria
clary sage

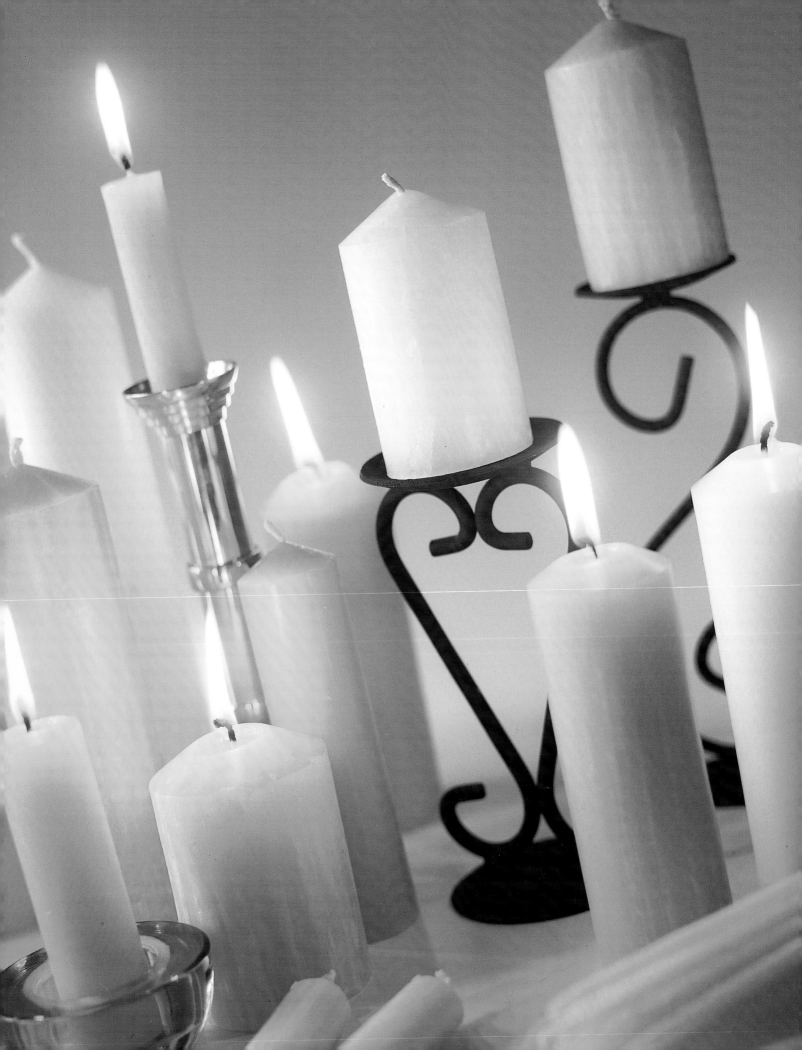

Sensual Scents

It is said that Cleopatra used the oils of jasmine and rose to woo Mark Antony.

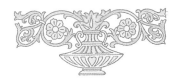

Legend has it that the Mogul prince, Jehangir, ordered roses to be floated in every canal in the royal gardens as he celebrated his wedding. His new wife ran her hands through the water and the gorgeous scent of the rose oil clung to her fingers. In tribute, Jehangir had the essential oils of roses extracted and bottled for his love.

There is a particularly exquisite group of essential oils — rose among them — that are known to be aphrodisiacs, some of them quite powerful. Use them creatively to put you in the mood and excite your senses. They can relax your mind and body (particularly if you are tired, stressed, or nervous).

Choose an oil or a combination of oils that particularly appeals to you and mix with a massage oil (see *Blending and Storing Oils* on page 24), then follow the guidelines in *Aromatherapy Massage* on page 28 for a luxurious full-body massage. Or rub the oil onto your body before slipping into a warm bath, either to prepare yourself or to share with a partner. You could drizzle a few drops of oil directly into the bathtub (make sure you disperse them before you get in). Candlelight and soft music can add to the mood. You can purchase special aromatherapy candles that are laced with essential oils which then linger in the air when burnt.

Fragrance a room with your chosen oils in a vaporizer, or an atomizer, or just sprinkle them around.

You can also annoint yourself with a heady perfume made from a blend of oils of your choice (see *Personal Perfumes* on page 58).

The "aphrodisiac" oils

Clary sage
sweet and uplifting, euphoria-producing

Geranium
floral, relaxing, uplifting

Jasmine
heady, luxurious

Neroli
deeply relaxing, dispelling anxiety and shyness

Orange
joyous, sensual, soothing

Patchouli
exotic, heady, sensual, soothing

Rose
romantic, heady, euphoria-producing

Sandalwood
exotic, spicy

Ylang ylang
relaxing, soothing

Oils for Beauty

While looking good begins with your inner health; your skin, hair and nails can all benefit from aromatherapy. There are essential oils to suit all skin and hair types, and they can be incorporated into a wide variety of treatments.

Essential oils may be called oils, but they are not oily. They are the diluted essences of plants.

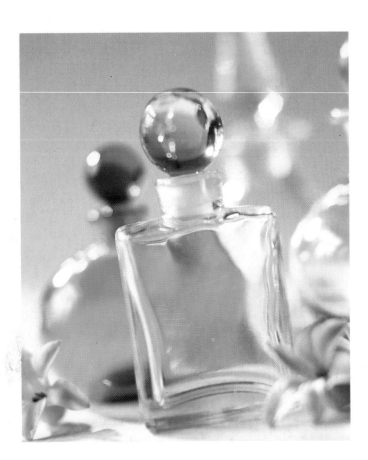

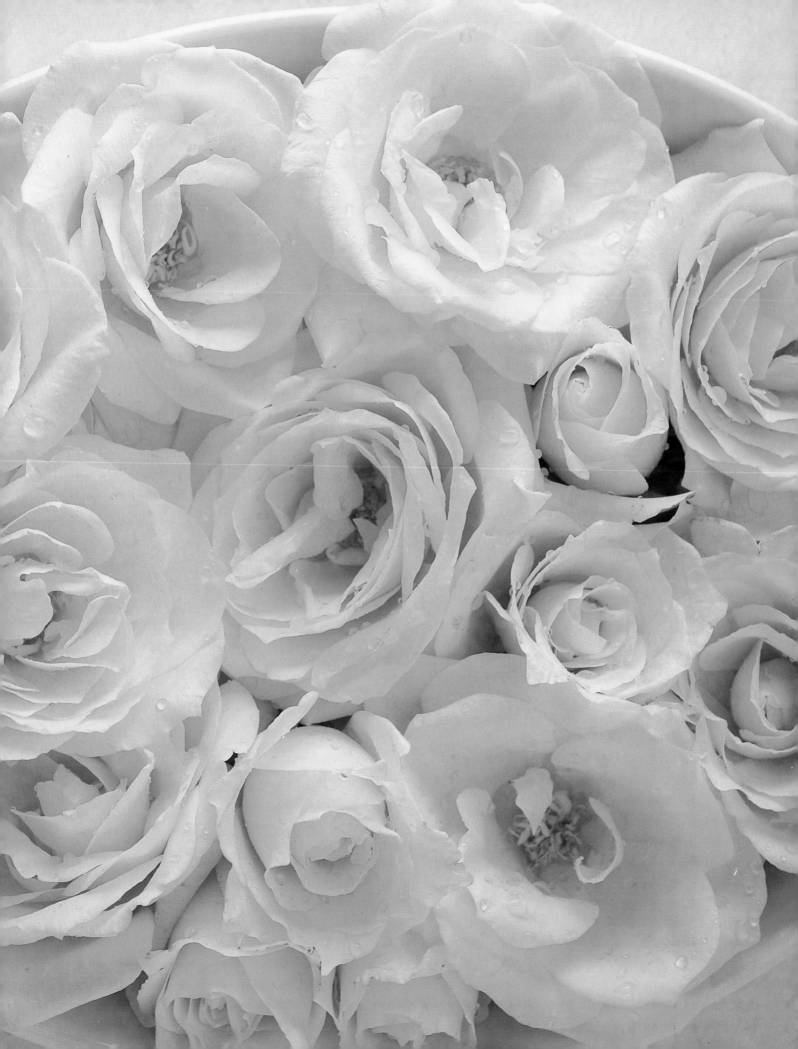

Facial cleansers

Select an essential oil or a blend suitable for your skin type from the list on page 50, and add a few drops to a mild, unperfumed cleanser or lotion available commercially.

Facial masks

Use clay, ground oatmeal, or a clay-base powder from a beauty supplier or pharmacist. Add hot distilled water and blend into a paste. Add 3 drops of your chosen essential oils to 1 teaspoon base powder, or 15 drops per cup of paste. Smooth the mix over your clean face, avoiding the skin around the eyes. Leave it to dry (about 10–15 minutes), then wash off with tepid water. For a smoother consistency, add plain yoghurt, and for very dry or sensitive skin add some jojoba, sweet almond, or vitamin E oil. Follow with a toner and moisturizer. Apply once a week to dry skin, and twice a week to oily skin.

Facial steaming

Steaming helps to hydrate, cleanse, and stimulate facial skin, and most skins benefit from a steam treatment every week or two. Cleanse your skin before you begin. Add 5–6 drops of essential oil to a large bowl of hot water, and drape a towel over your head and the bowl to prevent the steam from escaping. Steam for about 5 minutes to open pores, then wash your face with cool water. Follow with a toner and moisturizer.

Facial toners

Add a few drops of your chosen essential oils to an atomizer filled with distilled water. This will give you a spritzer that acts as a refreshing toner. A handy pocket-sized atomizer contains 2 oz (50 ml) water. Always use a glass atomizer, and shake well to disperse the oils. In summer, you may like to store the bottle in the refrigerator for a cool pick-me-up.

Facial moisturizers

The penetrative qualities of essential oils make them ideal nourishing treatments for softening the skin and making it supple and smooth. They will not clog up the pores and will help balance oily and inflamed skin.

If you prefer not to use base carrier oils (see page 26) as facial moisturizers, add a few drops of the essential oils for your skin type to a mild, unperfumed brand of moisturizing cream or lotion that contains mostly natural ingredients and not too many preservatives, dyes, and chemicals.

Toners are great for closing the pores of your skin. Use them on a piece of damp cotton to wipe your face and neck after cleansing or steaming or after masks. Avoid the eye area and make sure you choose a toner that suits your skin type.

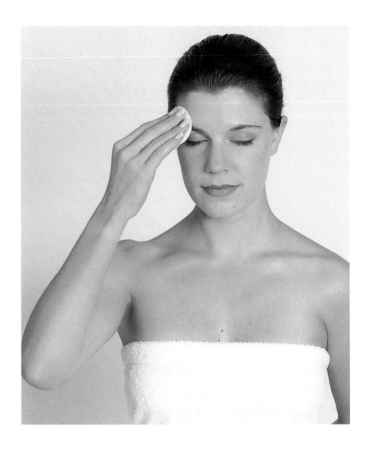

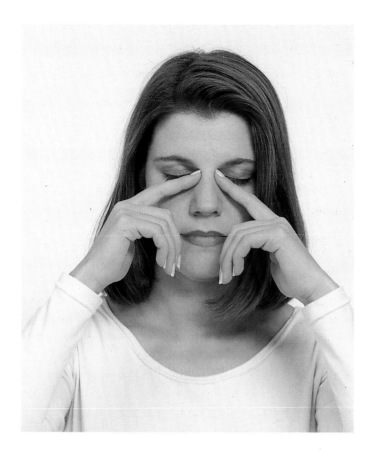
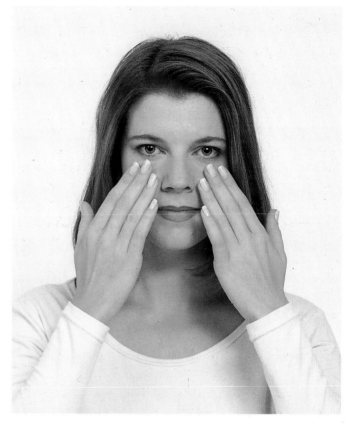

Facial massage

A facial massage can make you feel and look great. Try one as a special treat, or incorporate it into your weekly skin care regime for optimum benefits. Don't be too concerned about doing it "right"; whatever feels good will be beneficial. You should, of course, always be gentle as the skin on your face and neck is sensitive and you want to increase the circulation to help keep the skin firm, not stretch and pull at it.

Enhance the experience with your own special blend of essential oils added to a base carrier oil. Peach kernel oil is ideal as a base. Sweet almond oil can also be used, and jojoba oil is recommended for oily skin (see page 26). To 1 teaspoon base carrier oil, add 3 drops of a suitable essential oil selected from the list. Pour this mix into your hands and rub them together to warm them.

After cleansing, smooth the aromatherapy mix over your face and throat, avoiding the eye area. Make sure your hands are clean and be careful you do not scratch yourself with your nails. Try using the pads of your fingers, rather than the tips.

You may like to try some of these massage techniques, repeating each several times:

• Beginning with the pads of your thumbs in the middle of your forehead, stroke out to the temple area.

• Stroke along your jaw line from chin out to ears.

• Knead the chin area by gently squeezing and releasing along jaw line. Use your thumbs and fingers and work from the chin out to the ears.

• Try very gentle slapping to the cheeks and neck

• Smooth your fingers or palms across your cheeks and out to the ears

• Stroke over your eyebrows with your fingers

• Pinch along the eyebrows

• Squeeze along the edge of your ears

• With small circular movements, massage the mouth and cheek area

• Use small circluar movements to massage along the sides of your nose

• Using your index or middle fingers, press each side of the eyesocket at the top of the nose, and hold for several seconds.

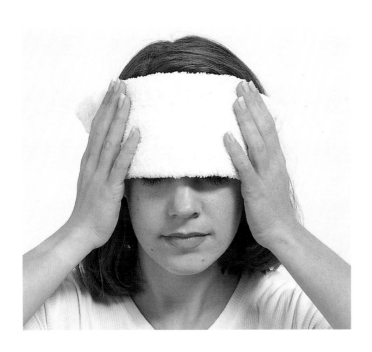

Compresses are particularly useful if base carrier oils are not at hand, or if your skin is oily or sensitive and irritated and you prefer not to use base carrier oils. A compress will refresh your skin. Use essential oils recommended for your skin type, and see page 22 for details on compresses.

Hand care

We often forget to pay attention to our hands, yet we expose them to harsh water, extreme temperatures, and damaging sunlight. Once a week or so, try to pamper them with an aromatherapy treatment.

1. Begin by soaking your hands in a bowl of lukewarm water to which a few drops lavender oil have been added. Dry them gently.

2. Exfoliate the skin to get rid of dead cells and soften hard skin: mix together 2 tablespoons raw sugar, 1 tablespoon base carrier oil, 2 drops lavender, and 2 drops lemon in a glass bowl, and rub into your hands before rinsing.

3. Follow with a moisturizing hand massage using 5 drops essential oils (those recommended for normal, dry, mature or sensitive skins) in 2 teaspoons base carrier oil.

4. To strengthen nails, make up a blend of 3 drops each lemon and lemongrass, and 2 drops each rosemary and lavender in 1 oz (30 ml) sweet almond oil, and rub a small amount into and around the nails and cuticles. Cypress and sandalwood are also good for the nails.

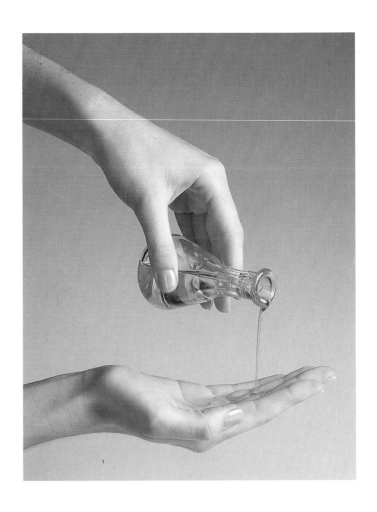

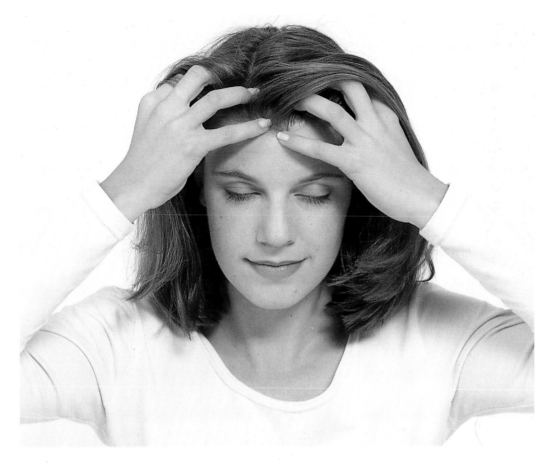

Essential oils for your hair type

Dry
cedarwood, sandalwood

Normal
lavender, chamomile

Oily
cedarwood, cypress, juniper, lavender, rosemary

Hair care

Cedarwood, clary sage, cypress, juniper, lavender, lemon, chamomile, rosemary, rosewood, and sage are all beneficial to the health of your hair.

Hair shampoo

Add 10 drops of essential oil suitable for your hair type (see lists above) to 15 oz (about 500 ml) of a natural, mild, unperfumed, non-detergent brand of shampoo or to shavings of pure soap dissolved in a bottle of water.

Hair rinses

To make a hair rinse for use after shampooing, choose an essential oil suitable for your hair type, or simply one whose perfume you will enjoy all day long. Then, depending on how strong you wish the scent to be, add 1–10 drops essential oil to 16 fl oz/500 ml water in a glass bottle. Shake well before using it as the final rinse after washing and conditioning. There's no need to rinse this mixture from your hair. If you have dark hair, you'll gain extra shine from rosemary, rosewood, or sandalwood. Fair hair will brighten with chamomile and lemon.

Intensive conditioning treatment

To improve the condition of your hair, use a warm oil treatment once a week to treat damaged hair, or once a month to pamper yourself. Jojoba oil is an excellent base carrier oil for hair treatments.

Make up a blend of 10–25 drops essential oils to 2–3 oz (60–100 ml) base carrier oil, depending on the length of your hair. Part your hair into sections. Apply the mixture along the sections all the way from the roots to the ends, with your fingers or absorbent cotton dipped in the oil. Wrap your hair in a warm towel, and try to leave the oil on for 2 hours for the best effect. If possible, sit in the sunshine or in a steamy bath. To remove, work in some shampoo and a small amount of water, then wash as normal.

Choose essential oils from those recommended for your hair type, or one of the following blends for particular hair problems:

For damaged hair, try a blend of geranium, lavender, and sandalwood.

For thinning hair, try lavender and rosemary.

For hair loss, try cedarwood and rosemary.

To strengthen hair, try bergamot, lavender, and rosemary.

Diluted essential oils make great natural deoderants. Try bergamot, cypress, lemon, tea tree, or sage for their clean scent and antibacterial properties.

Aromatherapy treatments for common beauty problems

Acne

Bergamot, camphor, chamomile, geranium, juniper, lavender, lemon, neroli, rose, sandalwood, tea tree, and ylang ylang are all recommended for acne, as these cleansing and antibacterial oils work as natural antiseptics and regulate the secretion of sebum. You can use them in the beauty preparations described in this chapter.

You can also try adding 5 drops each juniper and lemon oil to a basin of distilled, purified, spring, or mineral water. Soak balls of absorbent cotton in this mixture, squeeze them out gently, and then store the balls and the mixture in the refrigerator in separate airtight containers. When an outbreak of pimples occurs, wipe your skin every 2 hours with the cotton balls, and bathe your skin every night with the mixture. Or dilute 1 drop each chamomile and lavender oil on a damp cotton swab and apply to the pimple.

Bad breath

Add a drop of bergamot to a glass of water and gargle; do not swallow.

Cellulite

Mix together 4 drops juniper and 2 drops rosemary oil with 3 drops each cypress and patchouli in 6 teaspoons base carrier oil. Gently massage into the affected area every morning and night.

Dandruff

Massage the appropriate essential oil blend — see below — into your scalp and leave overnight. In the morning, shampoo your hair as usual. Use the mixture every second day until your dandruff is reduced.

For a dry, flaky scalp, add 4 drops each geranium, lavender, and sandalwood oil to 5 teaspoons base carrier oil such as sweet almond oil.

For an oily, scaly scalp, add 6 drops each rosemary and lemon oil to 5 teaspoons of a suitable base carrier oil such as jojoba oil.

Eye problems

For tired, irritated or puffy eyes, make a compress by soaking a cotton pad in a bowl of water to which chamomile, clary sage, lavender, or rose has been added. Wring out and place over your eyes, then rest for 10 minutes with eyes closed.

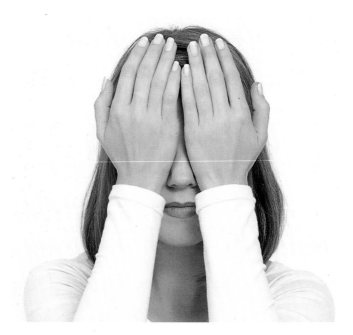

For relief from tired eyes, try rubbing the palms of your hands together until they are warm, then placing the palms or fingers over the eyes. Apply gentle pressure. You may like to incorporate this into an aromatherapy facial like the one on page 53.

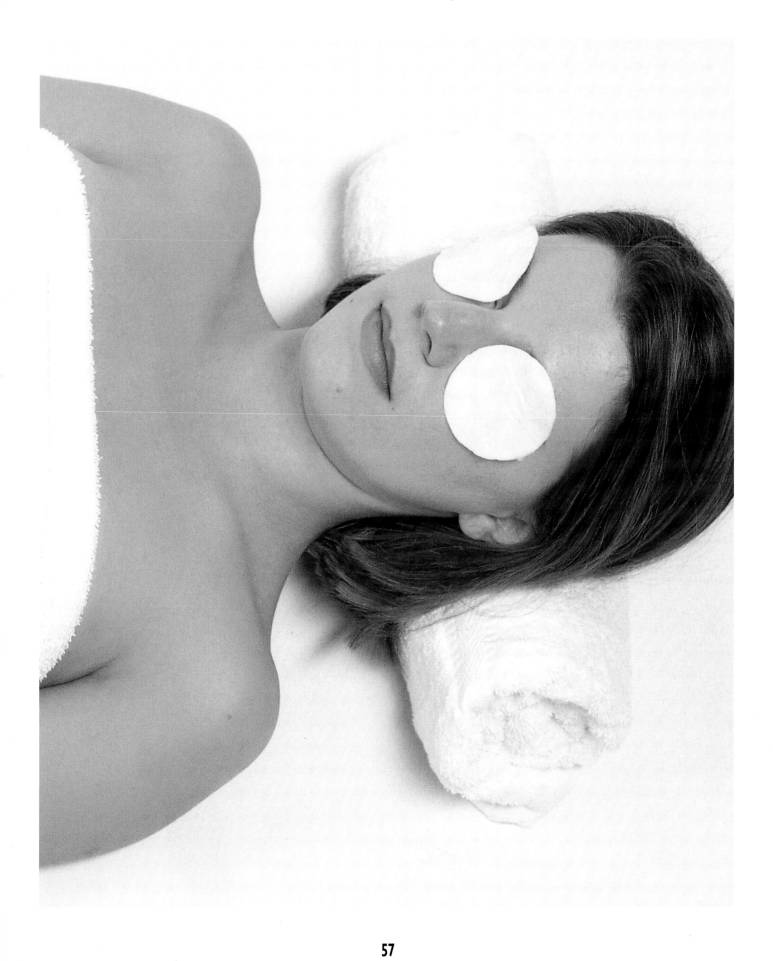

Personal Perfumes

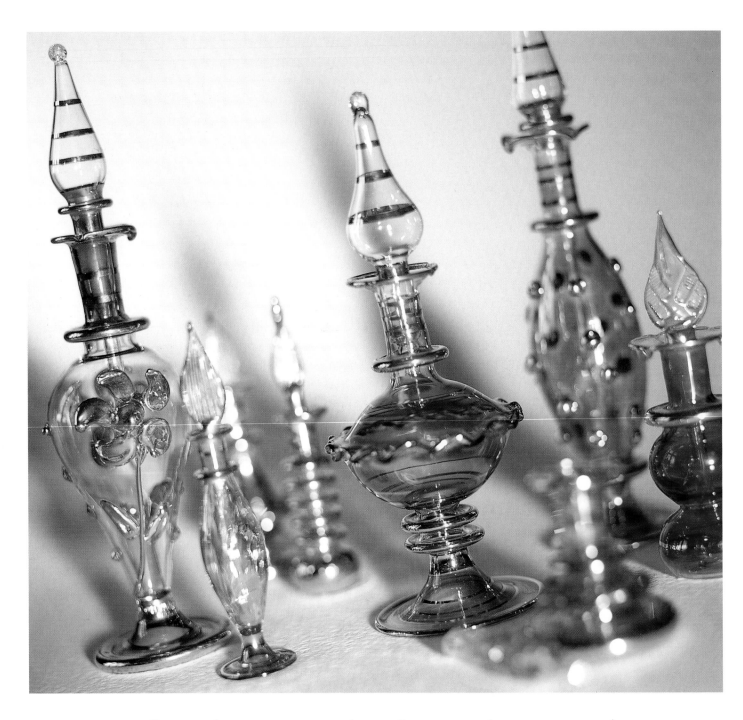

Remember — too much perfume can be overpowering,
so keep it subtle.

*M*any essential oils are admired for their gorgeous scent. You can make up your own individual blend of perfume to reflect your mood or the occasion. You may prefer a lighter perfume on hot summer days, while an exotic, heady scent can be perfect for a romantic evening.

Some of the essential oils that are most often used by perfumers are cedarwood, cinnamon, geranium, jasmine, lavender, neroli, orange, patchouli, and sandalwood.

Blending your perfume

If you are creating your own perfume, pure alcohol is the most efficient carrier, as it is clear and has no fragrance; it combines thoroughly with any essential oil, allowing for an even and light application. Once applied, the alcohol quickly evaporates, leaving no residue except the light, sweet scent of the chosen fragrance. If pure alcohol is not available, then a little vodka is a viable alternative, as it is the purest of the spirit beverages — another spirit might be sticky, stain clothes or skin, or have an unpleasant smell incompatible with essential oil fragrances. Jojoba oil also makes an ideal base as it will not oxidize and become rancid on the skin. For refreshing colognes, simply add your chosen essential oils to distilled or spring water, and shake vigorously.

Choosing the strength

The strength of your perfume will depend on the ratio of essential oil to the base oil, alcohol, or water. As a general guide, for perfume, use a 10% dilution, for eau de toilette, use a 5% dilution, and, for a splash cologne or atomizer spray, use a 1% dilution. You can use weaker blends in base carrier oils as body lotions, or add the essential oil to an unperfumed commercial body lotion.

A good place to start experimenting is by mixing together 2 teaspoons jojoba oil and 20 drops essential oil in a dark glass bottle, shaking the mixture, and then letting it stand for a few days in a cool, dark place so the oils will merge. If the mixture is too strong or overpowering for you, add more jojoba oil or some alcohol to the mix to make it more subtle.

A guide to scents

F l o w e r y
bergamot, geranium, neroli

M u s k y
*jasmine, patchouli, rose,
sandalwood, ylang ylang*

S w e e t
*cedarwood, neroli, rose,
rosewood*

S p i c y
*cedarwood, lemongrass,
rosewood, sandalwood*

R o m a n t i c
*geranium, lavender, rose,
rosewood, sandalwood*

S e n s u a l
*jasmine, patchouli, sandalwood,
ylang ylang*

Never rub perfume into your skin — this will "bruise" the scent. Apply it to your pulse points: the inside of your wrists, behind your ears and behind your knees. Your body heat will help the perfume develop.

Scented Rooms

Create atmosphere and increase your sense of well-being by using essential oils in your surroundings, whether at work or at home. Your choice of oils will depend on the result you wish to achieve, and there are a myriad of ways to put them to use.

To disseminate essential oils in a wider environment, vaporizers, atomizers and light-bulb rings can be used — see *Using Essential Oils* on page 20 for details. However, the fragrance of essential oils can be enjoyed without any extra equipment. Soak a piece of absorbent cotton in essential oil and place around a room or among clothing, to scent the air. For maximum effect, place the scented cotton somewhere warm, such as behind a heater, or sprinkle the oils directly on the logs of a fire.

Clothes and linen

You can surround yourself with a pleasing fragrance by perfuming your clothing and lingerie. Use the same perfume as the one you wear (see page 58) or try a drop of rose, jasmine, neroli, or ylang ylang oil in the final rinse water when you wash. Make sure the oil is well dispersed in the water and does not touch the cloth directly.

A drop of lavender, either in the final rinse or diluted and sprinkled directly on to the fabric, will impart a lingering aroma to bed linen that will help you sleep.

Towels will have extra freshness if you add 1 drop lemon oil to the rinse water, or sprinkle a drop in the clothes dryer.

Storage

A little cedarwood or patchouli oil will help protect clothes from moths, but use sparingly or the smell could be too heavy. Wipe out the inside of your drawers with a damp piece of absorbent cotton sprinkled with a few drops of these essential oils. Or you may choose to use your perfume oils instead.

You can also make perfumed drawer liners by sprinkling a few drops of your chosen essential oil onto lengths of thick parchment-style paper (wallpaper is ideal) cut to fit the insides of drawers.

Air fresheners

A drop or two of bergamot and lemon oil will freshen a room anytime. Use on a cotton pad or in an atomizer or a vaporizer.

Insect repellents

Use citronella, eucalyptus, lemongrass, or tea tree oil in a vaporizer or in candles to keep unwanted insects away. Diluted in base carrier oils, these oils can also be applied to exposed skin.

Create a mood

The various essential oils have different influences on mood and can help create atmosphere:

- to stimulate the mind: rosemary, sage, thyme
- to create a feminine aura: geranium, jasmine, rose
- to clear the mind for psychic healing: lavender, lemongrass, sandalwood
- for a healing atmosphere in a sick-room: bay, rose, thyme
- for meditation: frankincense, jasmine, lavender, ylang ylang
- to complement a special celebration, such as a wedding: jasmine, rose
- for a stimulating party atmosphere: clary sage, geranium, orange
- for Christmas: cedarwood, frankincense, myrrh, orange, pine, sandalwood
- for romance: patchouli, rose, sandalwood, ylang ylang

For the workplace

You can use the refreshing and uplifting essentials oil to promote motivation, decisiveness, and productivity. Basil, bergamot, juniper, lemon, peppermint, rosemary, and rosewood are particularly recommended.

The antiseptic and antibacterial oils will help prevent illness from spreading around the office; these include bergamot, eucalyptus, juniper, lavender, lemon, pine, and tea tree.

Refer also to *Treating Stress* on page 46.

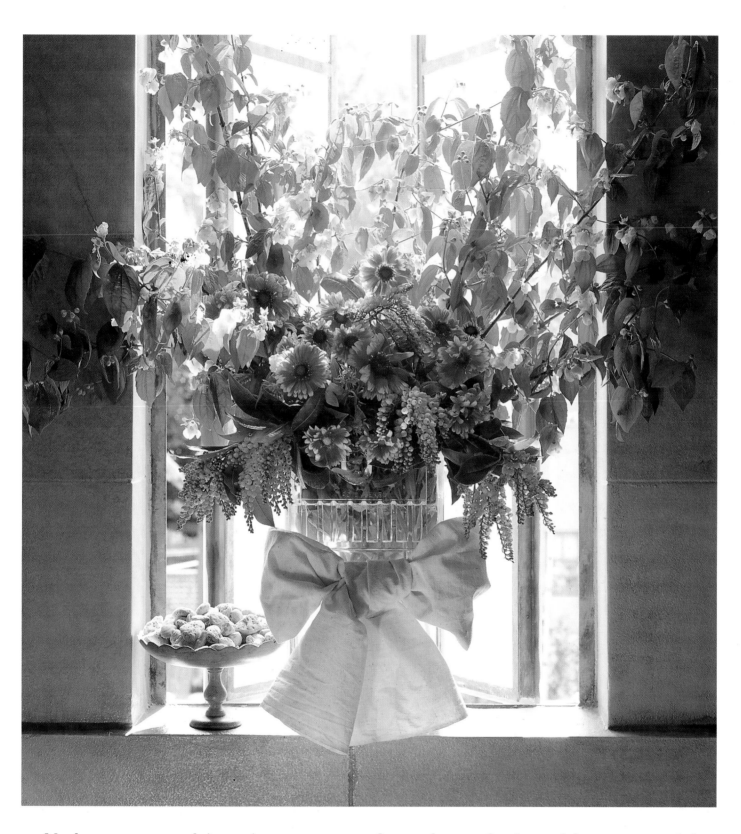

Make a personal imprint on a new home by replacing old aromas with your own blend of essential oils.

Index

Published by Lansdowne Publishing Pty Ltd
Level 5, 70 George Street, Sydney, NSW 2000, Australia
Chief Executive Publisher: Jane Curry
Publishing Manager: Deborah Nixon
Production Manager: Sally Stokes
Project Co-ordinator: Kirsten Tilgals
Project Assistant: Amalia Matheson
Project Consultant: Karen Bailey
Stylist: Mary-Anne Danaher
Photographer: André Martin
Designer: Michelle Wiener

First published in 1996
© Copyright: Lansdowne Publishing Pty Ltd

Set in Caslon 540 Roman on Quark Xpress
Printed in Singapore by Tien Wah Press (Pte) Ltd

National Library of Australia Cataloguing-in-Publication Data
The fragrant art of aromatherapy.
Includes index.
ISBN 1 86302 463 8.
1. Aromatherapy.
615.321

Photographic props and assistance lent by:
Grandma Goes Global, Paddington NSW Australia
House & Garden, Sydney NSW Australia
Jurlique, locations throughout Australia
Made on Earth, Sydney NSW Australia
Naturecare, Artarmon NSW Australia
Penelope Sach, Woollahra NSW Australia
Red Earth, locations throughout Australia
Roma Candles, Sydney NSW Australia
Sanctum, Byron Bay and Sydney NSW Australia
The Glass Stopper, Drummoyne and Surry Hills NSW Australia
The Fragrant Garden, Erina NSW Australia
Venustus, Paddington NSW Australia